D0955320

Presented To:

_____

From:

_____

Date:

_____

Kisses from

A
Good
God

DESTINY IMAGE BOOKS BY PAUL MANWARING

What on Earth is Glory?

Kisses
from

A
Good
God

XOXOXO

Accessing God's Intimate
Presence in Difficult Times

Paul Manwaring

DESTINY IMAGE₀ PUBLISHERS, INC.
P.O. Box 310, Shippensburg, PA 17257-0310
"Promoting Inspired Lives."

This book and all other Destiny Image, Revival Press, MercyPlace, Fresh Bread, Destiny Image Fiction, and

Treasure House books are available at Christian bookstores and distributors worldwide.

For a U.S. bookstore nearest you, call 1-800-722-6774.
For more information on foreign distributors,
call 717-532-3040.
Reach us on the Internet: www.destinyimage.com.

ISBN 13 TP: 978-0-7684-0309-1
ISBN 13 Ebook: 978-0-7684-8777-0
ISBN 13 HC: 978-0-7684-0322-0

For Worldwide Distribution, Printed in the U.S.A.

1 2 3 4 5 6 7 8 / 16 15 14 13 12

Dedication

This book is dedicated to the greatest kiss from God
that came in the season
about which this book is written.

To my first grandson,
Aidan James Manwaring
Before you were born, you changed history
and gave me a reason to fight.
Your birth marked the first time
three generations of Manwaring men
walked this earth together.
Since your birth, you have brought
greater joy and happiness than words can express.
I Love You, Aidan
Papa

Acknowledgments

This book is really one single acknowledgement of my family, friends, co-workers, surgeon, and, of course, an extravagantly good God who made this journey and story possible. I will never forget Bill Johnson's words as I finished preaching this message six weeks after having surgery: "Tonight we have heard our culture defined in the midst of suffering." As Bill said that, I stood next to his wife, Beni Johnson, who gave me the title for my message and subsequently, this book. "Call it 'Kisses from a Good God,'" she said. Thank you, Beni.

Since that day, so many have encouraged me to write this book. I am grateful for each one of you and for the testimonies I have received from those who were inspired on their journey by my original message.

Thank you to Bill and Ted for the two forewords. You both have different careers and ministries, and yet you are so alike in your absolute love for God and in the way you have encouraged and inspired me.

Three special women have helped with the manuscript. Chelsea Moore, who edited it for me with the challenge of correcting my grammar while protecting my voice. You have done a great job and are a true daughter in my life! Pam Spinosi, thank you for your ability to check the finest details. And Sue— for whom reading the manuscript was not easy—I needed your eyes to confirm that I had recorded the story accurately.

I cannot write these acknowledgements without naming my surgeon, Dr. Thijssen. Thank you for your skill, extraordinary bedside manner, and for the now 14 post-op appointments, providing us the opportunity to talk about cameras and share life.

And to my two sons, I am sure you know this already, but it is your daily love, sarcasm, and laughter—which you bring with occasional references to a kiss from a good God—that are my encouragement. And of course to Amy, my daughter-in-law, who will, by the time this book is published, have presented us with my second grandchild. Thank you for continuing to enrich my life.

And finally, to the One who has been misrepresented by so many. He really is a good God, and it's time that the whole world knew!

Endorsements

Kisses from a Good God is an extraordinary book full of encouragement and hope for those in the midst of great physical trials. I loved Paul's transparency, and the amazing God-given insights presented in the book will enable you also to walk through cancer, illnesses, and everyday life in total victory.

CAROL ARNOTT
Catch the Fire Ministries

I have traveled in my own Valley of the Shadow of Death. That journey led me to the table prepared in the presence of my enemies. Paul Manwaring's book made emotion fill my eyes—we are fellow travelers. His book helped me see the many "kisses" of God on my own path. Hospitals, doctors, nurses, and technicians are gloves that are filled by the healing hand of God. I applaud them! I encourage you to read the book, program your heart, receive good things from a good God, and He will be sure to make all things beautiful in its time! Beauty for ashes.

STEVE WITT

I'll never forget the day I took Paul to the doctor to get the results of his cancer tests. The nurse led us to a cold, white, sterile office, and seated Paul on the examining table. "The doctor will be in to see you in a few minutes," she said in a serious tone. I found a chair in the corner and sat down. The atmosphere was tense, so I tried to be funny to lighten the air. It seemed like we sat there for an eternity as we waited for the specialist. Finally, I heard the footsteps of the doctor grow louder as he neared the room. My heart began to race with anxiety as I anticipated the possible scenarios. The door opened and a tall, older man in a long white coat entered the room. I immediately knew that something serious was wrong by the stress on his face.

Without making eye contact, he began to give Paul his prognosis, using large, technical words and complex scenarios, almost as if he was hiding the bad news in some foreign language. Paul, being a former nurse, probably had some idea of what he was saying, but I was completely lost. I looked up at the doctor and said, "I'm sorry, but I didn't understand a word you said. Could you please say that again in plain English?"

"Your friend has prostate cancer," he explained in a monotone voice. "It's a level nine, which is the worst possible scenario."

Paul turned white as a ghost and looked as if he wanted to run out of the room. I scrambled to think of questions that might help breathe some hope into the situation, but the longer the doctor talked, the more critical Paul's condition seemed. We left the doctor's office in a daze, struggling to understand how to find God in this life-threatening test. After all, Bethel Church was famous for healings. We had seen thousands of miracles over the previous ten years. We intensified our prayer effort for Paul, but the miracle never came.

It wasn't that we didn't believe in doctors. After all, it was Jesus who said, "It's the sick who need a physician" (see Luke 5:31). It's just that we believe in miracles more. Weeks later, the operation took place, and shortly after we learned that Paul was cancer free!

Paul's recovery opened a door of revelation to us. We began to understand that miracles happen in different ways. Although God often heals people through prayer, there are other times the Great Physician chooses to co-labor with His medical interns to see wholeness restored to the life of His people.

If you are sick, or know someone who is, *Kisses from a Good God* is for you. It will bring hope to your soul, joy to your spirit, and healing to your body. You won't be disappointed!

KRIS VALLOTTON
Co-Founder of Bethel School of Supernatural Ministry
Author of eight books, including *The Supernatural Ways of Royalty* and *Spirit Wars*
Senior Associate Leader of Bethel Church, Redding, California

Rolland and I have had our faith in the goodness of God tested to the extreme over and over throughout our ministry. We identify with Paul Manwaring completely. And like Paul, we have learned to trust God without reserve, however He chooses to love us. We are after the outcome of His dealings with us, which is always more gracious and magnificent than we expect. Read this book to be encouraged all the more!

HEIDI BAKER, PhD
Founder and Director, Iris Global

Paul Manwaring is my dear friend and brother in the Lord. His new book *Kisses from a Good God* is a wonderful story of God's grace through the dark times in our lives. While his story refers to his battle with cancer, the truths stated in this book are relevant to every encounter we have with darkness in our lives. I have walked through my own dark times from accidents and recovery, through surgeries and healing. Each of these events has given me an upgrade and new supernatural authority in the areas the enemy attacked. This book is built on solid biblical principles, personal experiences, and practical applications that will both arm and protect you. Paul has been faithful to continue the testimony of Jesus, which is the spirit of prophecy. GET READY FOR YOUR UPGRADE!

LEIF HETLAND
President, Global Mission Awareness
Author of *Seeing Through Heaven's Eyes*

Paul writes as he lives: gentle, relaxed, disarming, profound, and inspiring everyone to greater things in God. *Kisses from a Good God* is not only an essential read for anyone going through any kind of trial, but for anyone who knows another human being! It is packed full of gems found in the kingdom.

As a veterinary surgeon, a Brit, and a pastor, having a resource that touches on the Father's heart, sonship, healing of life's hurts, friendship, science and medicine, and leadership is a natural gold mine. I believe in God's power. I believe in Him working through His kids, too. This book will not only encourage everyone who reads it, it will change lives,

attitudes, culture, and, therefore, the very environment you find yourself in.

STUART GLASSBOROW
Lead Pastor, Catch the Fire London

Contents

Foreword *by Ted Sawchuk* 23

Foreword *by Bill Johnson* 27

Introduction 31

Chapter 1   Ready or Not, Here I Come! 37

Chapter 2   Soul Management 47

Chapter 3   Gaps, Waits, and Journeys 55

Chapter 4   A Week of Kisses 65

Chapter 5   Encouraged by Heaven 75

Chapter 6   Saved by a Dream 83

Chapter 7   A First-Class Healing 95

Chapter 8   He Really Is Good 105

Chapter 9   Shine the Light 115

Chapter 10   Family: God's Big Idea 125

Chapter 11   Restored Fortunes 133

Chapter 12   Become a Kiss 149

Chapter 13   Whispering Shame 159

Chapter 14   Re-Sign 171

Afterword 181

Foreword

by Ted Sawchuk

I'm honored to write a foreword for Paul Manwaring's new book, *Kisses from a Good God.* Paul is a dear friend I met because of the message he shared in this book. Most forewords in Christian literature are written by ministers and theologians. I am neither. I am a physician and a surgeon. I specialize in urology. Taking care of patients with prostate cancer is what I do daily.

I grew up in a Charismatic home, where praying for the sick and believing them to be healed was the norm. My father, a family physician, would come home with stories about praying for patients and seeing God move in their lives. He was part of my inspiration for going into medicine. My family vacations growing up were often spent on medical missions. In medical school, I would eagerly attend Saturday morning lectures on embryology and be amazed at how God knit the human body together. I saw Psalm 139:13-14 come alive: *"For You created my inmost being; You knit me together in my mother's womb. I praise You because I am fearfully and wonderfully made; Your works are wonderful, I know that full well"* (NIV).

In residency training, I learned how to treat urologic diseases, both medically and surgically. Often, I would pray with patients for their surgery and treatments. I saw God move in people's lives. In practice, I continued to pray daily for my patients and often with them for successful outcomes. I could see God moving in patients. It seemed like God was doing His thing with healing and I was doing what I knew medically to see people healed.

I listened to a podcast in May of 2008 from Bethel Church by Paul Manwaring. He was talking about his ordeal with prostate cancer in a message called, "Kisses from a Good God." Naturally, as a urologist, listening to a pastor talk about prostate cancer was intriguing. Paul struggled with the same questions I have always had as a physician who believes in supernatural healing. I wondered why some were healed instantaneously and others needed to go through surgery and treatments to get better. When Paul talked about surgery and medicine not being a second-class healing and God touching him supernaturally through every step of his ordeal, it changed the way I viewed medicine and my profession. That simple message was probably the most profound pearl of wisdom that I have learned in all my years of training and practice.

We know that God answers our prayers and wants to see us healed. How He answers our prayers and how He heals us may be different than what we expected, but He is faithful! *Kisses from a Good God* should be read by any believer going through an illness or any trial of life. You will recognize how good our God is in all circumstances. I have given CDs of Paul's message to patients in the past. I am now excited to be able to recommend his book. *Kisses from a Good God* changed the way I view my medical practice. I know it will touch the reader's life in a similarly profound way.

TED SAWCHUK, MD
North Dakota

Foreword

by Bill Johnson

*K*isses from a Good God is about Paul Manwaring's extraordinary journey of faith. Abiding
faith is the glowing ember of the heart that explodes
into a fiery display of God's vengeance against the
enemy afflicting us. This is not the kind of faith that
seems almost faddish, which for some has become
the magic pill that fixes everything. This kind comes
from encountering and knowing the One who is *per-
fectly faithful*. Faith comes from relationship. It is
the offspring of the love of God. Perhaps that's what
the apostle Paul was describing when he said, "Faith
works through love" (see Gal. 5:6). Faith flows easily
from the heart of the one who knows he is loved.

Bad news has hit all of us at one time or another.
I wish it were avoidable. While I don't believe preparing for bad news is viable for the believer, I do
believe abiding in the love of God is. Love conquers
fear. The author's profound discovery of the goodness of God and His perfect love even in the midst of
adversity puts this wonderful story into a context that
everyone can follow. This is *mission possible*.

Look at these verses:

> **And not in any way terrified by
> your adversaries, which is to them
> a proof of perdition**, *but to you of
> salvation, and that from God* (Philip-
> pians 1:28 NKJV).

> *In righteousness you shall be estab-*
> *lished; **you shall be far from***
> ***oppression, for you shall not fear;***
> *and from terror, for it shall not come*
> *near you* (Isaiah 54:14 NKJV).

Winning the fear war is crucial. Every time we do, we send shock waves into the realms of darkness, reminding them of their end and of our ongoing victory through Christ! Paul Manwaring describes in detail how that war is to be won in the battleground of our minds.

Thankfully, this book does not try to provide a "one size fits all" formula to the problems of life. Paul goes much deeper than that, setting us on a pathway of personal discovery, personal encounter. He bears his soul, allowing us to see his journey without hype and fluff. This is the real deal.

I much prefer instant breakthrough to a drawn-out process. But where faith brings an answer, enduring faith brings an answer with character. Paul's testimony is a profound example of the breakthrough that comes through saying yes to a process. And now the rich reward of God has been given to his family.

The Manwaring victory has become a corporate blessing for us at Bethel Church. Through this book, countless thousands will become equipped to turn potential tragedy into triumph, bringing individuals and entire families into great victory.

Paul Manwaring is one of the most authentic believers I know. He walks his talk every day of his life, with unwavering devotion to Christ and his family. He has an uncompromising resolve to fulfill his assignment on this planet. One of my greatest privileges is to work with him and see the hand of God upon him—I am amazed. I commend the man and his message.

BILL JOHNSON
Bethel Church
Author, *When Heaven Invades Earth*
and *Essential Guide to Healing*

Introduction

I was diagnosed with prostate cancer in 2008 at the age of 50. I doubt I would have written a book on this subject were it not for the encouraging response to my sermon, "Kisses from a Good God," which I preached on May 2, 2008, just six weeks after my surgery to remove the cancer. I made a statement in that message that would birth a relationship with a doctor who performs as many as 35 prostatectomies a year. As I shared my story, I confidently stated that surgery is not a second-class healing. It was such a simple remark, but one that had a life-changing impact on my friend, Dr. Ted Sawchuk.

Two months after my surgery, I stood in the kitchen of another doctor friend of mine and we talked about healing. He said to me that the goal is to get well. He told me that if I had a headache, he would pray for me. If the headache remained, he would give me a pain reliever. Why? Because the goal is to get well. My journey to get well took me to the operating room. Yes, I would have preferred a dramatic, supernatural intervention. But strangely, I now enjoy the fruit of a journey I did not choose to take.

Kisses from a Good God is my journey through one of the toughest seasons of my life. Many others have written their stories of life's trek through difficult seasons, and I am honored to join the ranks. For certainly every account of a journey through suffering is written down to encourage our fellow travelers. God's ability to take the worst things and turn them to good is so extraordinary that we often mistakenly believe that He must have sent the worst of it. The outcome of His hand on our lives is always so profound that we can wrongly think He must have planned it all, even the struggle.

The dilemmas that we face can be summed up in Psalm 77:10: *"Then I said, 'It is my grief, that the right hand of the Most High has changed.'"* It often feels when we are presented with challenges that it is God who has changed or moved. But the opposite is the case: it is our grief, our changed perspective, which causes our view of God to change. I suggest that it is not just grief, but every other thing that can shift our perspective and alter our view of God. In the midst of trial, we may perceive that He is silent or not doing anything, but that is unlikely to be the case. This is my story of facing a challenging circumstance, but with a good God. Each chapter was written with the hope that it will be the message you or someone you love needs to hear on their journey through life's challenging circumstances.

Soon after I shared this story from the pulpit for the first time, I received an e-mail from a woman who had listened to the message while sitting in an oncologist's waiting room. In the e-mail, she wrote that as she listened, she felt that someone who understood was there with her. It was that kind of encouragement which also motivated me to write this book. I will also never forget the moment when a very successful doctor sat next to me, a woman with years of training and experience, and told me that I had changed the way she practiced medicine. It was both humbling and shocking, and yet another reason to write my story.

My surgery took place over Easter weekend, 2008, and included a near death experience. I quipped at the time, "Jesus went to hell at Easter, but He came back with keys." I then declared that I wanted my keys. Little did I know what they might be. Now, however, I know that one key was to be invited into a place of influence in my beloved world of healthcare. A career I left nearly 30 years ago has opened its doors to me again. And as I write this introduction, I am returning home from a conference where doctors shared their case studies of miraculous healings. I was honored to be there and listen to my friends share their victories, these friends who daily live out the interplay of the supernatural with the skills they learned in medical school. At the end of the meeting, these doctors, nurses, and even hospital administrators formed the ministry team and prayed for the sick. It was a historical moment. These healthcare professionals, of all people, know what they are praying for and whom they pray to: Creator God, whose name and nature is Healer.

This is my story, but it is no longer mine alone. It is a journey that is shared by those who are on their own healing passage, walking someone else through the battle of disease, or facing some other type of crisis, all of which can, in a moment, change our lives forever. I am certain that the content of this book can be applied to countless of life's circumstances.

I believe that the profound is sometimes communicated through the simplest of things: a timely e-mail from a friend, a phone call, or a spontaneous prayer. And so it is my hope and prayer that as you read each chapter, simple messages will be released as though they were written just for you. May you experience the moments along the way when something simple—something someone says or does, or something that you read—can be for you like a kiss from a good God.

Chapter 1

Ready or Not, Here I Come!

"Nothing can prepare you." This is a phrase that invited itself to become part of my vocabulary the minute some of life's worst news invaded my world. But it was simply not true.

I have heard these words muttered so many times in the aftermath of a tragedy or the delivery of bad news. While true for some, the idea that nothing can prepare you is not universally applicable. Of course, the presence in my life of the unwelcome visitor, cancer, did creep up on me by surprise. All of the sudden, the trespasser I had seen in so many others' lives invaded my world, and with that certainly comes shock. But was I unprepared? No!

I increasingly believe that the mask of being unprepared is just this: a subtle mind game played by the enemy of our souls to prevent us from accessing the experiences and lessons that have prepared us for such events. It is a lie that suggests that no one else has been on the journey that we are about to travel. It is a lie that will effectively prevent us from building relationship with those who have walked through similar circumstances and won authority along the way. It is an invitation to a lonely walk with self-pity as a willing traveling companion, diverting us from the strength available in those around us. Had I believed that nothing had prepared me, I would have entered an abyss of self-pity and, in that place, potentially missed the strength that was available to me.

Wherever we live, we exist within a culture. Simply put, a *culture* comprises the practices and traditions by which we cope with our world. The notion of unpreparedness is a manifestation of a culture that addresses crises outside of relationship with a good God. We sometimes create a culture to protect ourselves from a certain environment. For instance, in Spain, realizing that the fiercest rays of the sun are at noon and the two hours following, the culture established the *siesta*—shutting down for a few hours in the afternoon—to protect the people from the heat of the sun.

I suddenly had to ask myself: What culture will this invading cancer land in? What will grow in the medium of my life, and what beliefs and practices will protect me from earth's fierce cancerous rays? Am I prepared? Can anything prepare me? The truth is, I was prepared, and I believe that many who read this book were also prepared for such moments in life. The question is, more correctly: Do I have the ability to access what has been put inside of me and around me for such a time as this?

Shortly after I received the news of cancer invading my body, I realized that many people and circumstances had already prepared me—most significantly, both my wife and best friend, who immediately rallied around me and poured strength into my life. My bad news also fell into the context of my past experience as a trained nurse. I have been present in many different scenarios and watched as the difficult news of cancer was delivered to a patient. I have also heard the many testimonies of cancer healed, both supernaturally and with the aid of medicine and surgery. The question then becomes this: Which of these experiences and memories do I attach my thoughts and emotions to? If I am surrounded by a culture that blames God, I will do the same, and in the process shut down my access to His goodness. I will still be relating to God, but it will be through a lens that misrepresents Him, a lens that says He sends cancer.

Besides the people in your life, the culture surrounding you will also contribute to your level of preparedness. When I was diagnosed, I had lived for over six years in a community that is founded on the understanding of the goodness of God. In this culture, the behavior of the people reinforced the teaching that God is good, creating in me and many others the ability to access His goodness even in the midst of things that we do not understand. Now I hope to stand in the place of helping you prepare for or walk through your fire—although my prayer is that the fire never comes.

As the unsolicited word *cancer* entered my world, I knew that the word itself would create a culture of its own and—as with many sicknesses and crises—consume "normal" life with its insatiable appetite.

What used to be normal would be replaced by a new normal: hospital visits, blood tests, specialists who discuss options and introduce a new language that would appear across the landscape of life for the coming days, weeks, or months. The degree to which this new normal takes over life depends on the nature of the disease, the severity, and the treatment options. However small or large the cultural shift is, as this new normal is introduced—especially in the case of cancer—a cloud enters the atmosphere of the victim and perhaps, more importantly, that of his or her family.

The fear of death is bad enough, but the robbery that takes place on the way to death is often the more painful to watch and be part of. I well remember, as a nurse, the first cancer patient in my care. He was *barrier nursed* at the London Hospital, Whitechapel, which meant that his "normal" required all of his visitors to wear masks, gowns, and gloves to prevent him from contracting infection, which could end his life. He lived in a cold, unfriendly world. As I cared for him one day, he told me that exactly a year before he had been given one year to live. Dates become so important and memorable on such a journey. Because of that, and the lack of any hope from the treatment he was receiving at the time, he told me that he wanted to go home. His desire was to have some "normal" in the last days of his life. If this was his end, then he wanted to decide how to spend it. For him, this meant abandoning the unfriendly and cold world of masks, gowns, and gloves. He wanted, instead, to hold his wife and kids and not be clinically isolated from those he loved and who loved him.

The discussion with the doctors that followed was not perhaps my finest hour as a nurse. It was, however, one of my early attempts to push back the culture of cancer and give some "normal" back to my patient. When addressing the doctors, I spoke not so much as a nurse, but as a son who had watched his father die of cancer. I spoke as a son who was holding on to some precious memories of moments by my father's bedside in our family home. I wanted my patient's family to experience what I had. Last words, last thoughts, last hugs—if death is the coming result—are so important. I was criticized by the doctors for my outspoken views and reminded that I was a mere student nurse. But one thing I knew: my patient was going home to "normal"!

As normal is challenged and the unwelcome imposter starts to dominate the culture in our lives, can we access what has prepared us to create a counterculture—an environment in which nourishing thoughts and feelings can grow rather than unhealthy ones fester and multiply? I particularly like the definition of *culture* as "the software of the mind, the default to which we return after any malfunction."[1] Familiar as most of us are now with computers, we know that *default* means that we can adjust a word-processing document, change fonts and margins, but that despite any changes we make, the default setting returns us to our most familiar page format. It lines up with the original standard. A culture that embraces the goodness of God needs to become so much a part of our lives, our thinking, and our habits, that no matter what adjustments take place, we have a default of His goodness to return to. This should be our "normal."

As Kris Vallotton, associate pastor at Bethel Church, teaches, if you have something on the lens of your eyeglasses, then whatever you look at will have the same flaw. If you have a flawed view of God, that flawed perspective will affect everything you look at. Your core values are influenced not by what you see, but how you see. The goal of our lives is to develop core values based on a true and healthy view of God and then live out those core values, creating heaven's culture on earth—a culture in which only the fruit of heaven can grow and mature, and the fierce and harsh rays of the enemy are not enabled to burn us with the sunburn of hell.

Our goal is to create a culture into which the unwelcome visitor—cancer, or other diseases and crises—may descend, but not survive. Cancer may shout, "Ready or not, here I come!" But when it does, it will be seen through a lens that says, "God cannot have sent it, it will not rob me of my identity, I am prepared, the price has been paid, I will be healed, heaven's culture will surround me, others have traveled this way before, and their victory will be my victory!" I am not saying it will be easy, but I do speak as a fellow traveler, and what's more, a victor.

Hell may shout, "Ready or not," but the good news arrives in heaven's reply. Heaven's number one representative has already come and is ready and waiting. For six months prior to my diagnosis of cancer, I had stomach problems. I was fairly convinced that it was lactose intolerance, but when the pain persisted, I decided to go and visit our family doctor. I had, by then, worked out that I had a parasite, and as my family doctor ordered the tests, I said, with a degree of self-confident bravado, "Test me for everything; I am 50 next week." I really don't go to the doctor very often and am blessed with good health. While I should have them more regularly, this was the first time that I was willing to have a full checkup. And so I had a blood test on my 50th birthday. It was, I know, a crazy way to celebrate, but I wanted to get rid of my parasite. The truth is, that parasite saved my life. It was perhaps my best birthday present ever.

Heaven was waiting and, I believe, revealed the news of cancer in my body, knowing that everything was prepared in order for me to deal with this situation. Hell screamed, exposed by a parasite, and heaven said, "Ready," even if I was, perhaps, not quite so quick.

Endnote

1. This definition was introduced by Geert Hofstede in his book *Cultures and Organization: Software of the Mind.*

Chapter 2

Soul
Management

So another of life's journeys began. I gave my blood on my birthday and shortly after that, headed off alone on a trip to Fresno, California. I had found myself living in California as a result of my wife's visiting Bethel Church, in Redding in August of 1999, to pursue her own desire for freedom and purpose. Moving to California was truly a step of faith, as back then few had heard of Bethel or Bill Johnson. There were no books, CDs, or websites. So much has changed since then. My wife's desire to be in Redding spawned a life-changing and, as I was about to find out, likely life-saving decision.

Journeys have become part of the Manwaring family culture. Emotional, spiritual, and even practical journeys have become our way of life. It was very different back in 1999. Before that point Sue had never been on a plane. The first flight she would ever take was an 11-hour flight from London to San Francisco. She still doesn't enjoy flying, but she travels the world to minister, and absolutely nothing will stop her flying when our grandson Aidan is waiting at the other end. Journeys are our way of life—although we don't always know where we are heading. Sometimes our journeys contain the unexpected, whether for good or whether as an obstacle. But as my boys will frequently tell me in our facetious family way, "It's all part of the journey, Dad."

Two days after my birthday, while in Fresno, I received an e-mail from my doctor saying that my PSA was 4.4. Not too much to worry about, he thought. However, despite his lack of concern, I began to worry. Sue and I have lived around the medical world long enough, and although we were a few hundred miles apart when the e-mail arrived, we both knew that it was not likely to be good news.

I was in Fresno to teach a Strategic Planning Workshop for a group of believers who were purposing to see their city transformed. We were meeting in a room with a clear view of the city, which in itself, felt strategic, not to mention that the assembled group included the future mayor of Fresno. The group consisted of personal friends of mine and I wanted to be there. I wanted to be there, that is, until the news arrived from my doctor. I mostly managed to bury my thoughts and emotions as I taught my way through the afternoon. But I no longer had anything to distract me as I returned to my hotel room, alone, with potential bad news spinning around in my head. In my room, I sat on my bed, knowing that in an hour I would be heading for dinner with some of my favorite church leaders; but I can assure you that I did not want to be with them on that occasion.

What do you do at times like that? I asked myself a question: *What would Bill Johnson do or teach others to do?* And then I recalled Bill saying at one time, "When you've lost your peace, open the book of Psalms and read it until you find your voice." Up until that point I had always viewed that as simply a good tip. We listen to teachings over and over; then we realize on the umpteenth time, "Oh, you mean to actually do that." Open the Psalms and read until you find your voice.

So, sitting cross-legged on a hotel bed, I opened my Bible to Psalms and began to read. I knew those early psalms well, yet I read them as if for the first time. In Psalm 4:3, it says, *"The Lord hears." Wow*, I thought, *the obvious can be so encouraging*. That is truly good news. I don't know if you realize just how good that news is, that He hears when you call to Him. Despite the encouragement that one line brought, I knew it was not the voice that I was looking for, so I read on. *Would I be here long?* I wondered. Maybe the great Psalm 119 would contain my voice?

But then it happened as I got to Psalm 13:2, *"How long shall I take counsel in my soul?"* Immediately, I saw that my soul is not a good counselor. That was it. Paul Manwaring, who is able to work nearly everything out with a nursing, management, and strategic background, had to know on that day that his soul, mind, will, and emotions could not be trusted as the primary guides for this journey. As I read on, Psalm 16 reminded me that my soul has the capacity to take me to Sheol or hell. *"For You will not abandon my soul to Sheol,"* reads Psalm 16:10.

My mental wanderings were already dragging me to the place where there is no hope and no answers, just more distress. In the hotel that day, I decided, between God and myself, that I would not study the PSA test result or anything related to it. I wouldn't go surfing the Net or even searching my soul. I would, as I went on to read in Psalm 16:7, *"Bless the Lord who has counseled me,"* and allow my mind to instruct me in the night season. The journey from Psalm 13 to Psalm 16 would be a journey I would take many times over in the coming months. It would prove to be a life-giving journey, a passage into the counsel of heaven.

I sat on the bed that day and thought, *It works, Bill, it really does!* There is, in this great book of Psalms, biblical instruction that has led me to spiritual and practical breakthrough. That day, my soul was discharged from any responsibility to counsel me, and from then until my surgery, that advice from the psalmist—written thousands of years earlier—became my personal lifeline. I discovered that my own view of reality is a rather poor counselor. My view of what test results may or may not mean, and my ability to chew over every wild, negative thought that entered my head were not going to counsel me out of my situation. I had decided not to look anything up on the Internet about my condition, and I stuck to that. In fact, I took it to a slight extreme, as on one occasion I sat in the doctor's office for over an hour and refused to read any of the books on his shelf. I wouldn't even pick them up. I was not going to allow my mind to be filled with the fear-inflicting possibilities of cancer. I couldn't afford to because I knew myself, and those facts and information would cause me to spin out of control, providing open doors for thoughts to rush in. I am sure I don't have it completely right and I'm not saying I didn't ever have a negative thought enter my mind. My wife Sue knows the truth of the matter. What I do know is that the Psalms helped me to manage my thoughts in a way I would have been incapable of without their truth.

There is an amusing aspect to this part of my journey. On several occasions I had to spend time in the examination room waiting for my doctor to come and examine or counsel me. I sat in a room surrounded by charts, illustrations, and models of parts of the human anatomy. There were also several books in the office, books which I had vowed not to read during this season. As I glanced at their titles, I was amused, and to be honest, a little offended that one of them was called *Prostate Cancer for Dummies*. *Really*, I thought, *this disease shouldn't be treated so lightly*. What kind of heartless person would give a book about prostate cancer the kind of title that I was used to seeing on books about computers and photography? I chose not to say anything about the book to my doctor.

The day of my diagnosis, I sat in the doctor's office with two of my best friends. During the awkward wait, I happened to mention the book for dummies, telling them my degree of humorous insult. We laughed as I said, "What kind of person would tell the unwilling victims of this disease that they are dummies?" After my diagnosis had been given to me and a plan for prayer and surgery was established, the doctor, in a completely unsolicited statement, announced that of all the advice he could give me, he would highly recommend that I consult with his favorite book. Yes, you've guessed it! I am sure it is a very good and helpful book. We all laughed—probably a great vent after the diagnosis—and had to explain the joke to the doctor. For the record, I never did read the book. I had some far better advice from an old psalmist!

I have watched so many times as others lose sight of life and all of its promises, allowing their mind, will, and emotions to govern their decisions. By His grace, that day in Fresno, I found a way out. We live in an age of which the previous generation only had a glimpse. At any moment, we can listen to news from around the world or search any subject on the Internet. It is an incredible age that also comes at a price. God gave me permission to live through this season of my life in a degree of isolation from our constant access to information. It was not because I do not value advice and medical knowledge. But for a time, I received my advice from God, which enabled me to more easily access the things that He wanted to speak to me, whether through His word, His voice, His people, or any other method.

As you face the situations in your own life and ask yourself how to move forward, you will have to find the answer for yourself. It will vary from person to person and depend on background and existing knowledge or experience. But I can offer no better advice for a point of crisis and loss of peace than to read the Psalms until you "find your voice."

Chapter 3

Gaps, Waits, and Journeys

The Bible is a wonderful work of literature, history, biography, and the acts of God. Despite the Bible's profound content, sometimes what it *doesn't* say teaches us most. There are an abundance of unmentioned facts and details throughout the Bible. These can be discovered in the questions we are left asking and the areas where we are left wanting. Who was that character? Why was she so little mentioned? How long did she have to wait before her life changed for the better? These are, for me, the gaps, waits, and journeys.

Pondering the unspoken details of the Bible is a rich resource for learning the journey of faith. My reading of Genesis 12 and the example of faith expressed within the book influenced my own journey from England to America. In this context, I did not come across the passage by chance; but I was traveling to work one day in 2001 when I asked God for a biblical example that would encourage me as Sue and I led our family into the unknown. All I heard Him say was, "Genesis chapter twelve." With hindsight, His answer was obvious: Genesis 12 is the story of a man leaving the land of his fathers and going on a journey to another country.

When I got to work that day in 2001, I immediately read Genesis 12. The details of that passage were so clear as I read of a place called Bethel, which was east of the mountains, and even the mention of giant trees. It was as if Northern California was in the Bible. For those who do not know, mountains to the north, west, and east surround Bethel Church. And on the coast—just 150 miles west of Redding—are the giant redwood trees.

However, the Bible doesn't give us the details of Abraham's journey, although I am sure there were cold, lonely, and frightening moments. Despite the lack of details, Abraham's story is a reference point for all of us who are called to and follow a life of faith. Faith and the unknown are essential companions; otherwise, we can no longer call it *faith*. Abraham shows us that it is the journey *of* faith—not arriving at a destination—that attracts heaven's attention. Hebrews 11:8 reads, *"By faith Abraham, when he was called, obeyed by going out to a place which he was to receive for an inheritance; and he went out, not knowing where he was going."*

I look forward someday, although not too soon, to learning the histories of the obscure biblical characters, the ones whose journeys aren't given in full detail, the ones who had to wait. Our Bible is understandably condensed, and it is easy to read the stories without embracing the waits. We humans can be so impatient. We have the ability to travel thousands of miles in a matter of hours, yet we consider an extra hour or two layover in a comfortable airport to be disastrous. The heroes of our faith knew no such luxuries, and, as we read, their layovers could be as long as 40 years.

When it came to my journey with cancer, there were to be several waits along the way. One-hour waits in the examination room, wondering if the doctor had forgotten me—thankful for an iPhone to occupy me as I kept to my no soul-searching agreement and ignored the books and charts which filled the room. Then there were the days following the biopsies, the wait for surgery, the first pathology, and the following blood tests, which accompany me for a full five years after the surgery.

Our globalized, fast food, instant communication world has trained us to be impatient. Waiting is no longer a way of life for the Western civilized world. Strawberries that used to be enjoyed during a short summer season are now available year-round. Let it be known that you can never beat a naturally ripened and freshly picked English strawberry (perhaps with some clotted cream as you watch Wimbledon tennis).

The truth is, the waits are realities. Every one, for me, was an individual challenge giving me a choice of what to fill my thoughts with. What we fill our minds with while we wait will be, for all of us, the ultimate challenge. But my counselor, the book of Psalms, prepared me well. For some of the waits, I was able to leave my desk and go to the prayer chapel on the Bethel campus. For others, I would make myself busy; and for some, I had to find a way to press through just so I could go to sleep at night. He is a faithful God, and in my wife He gave me a companion who would walk with me. And together we would remind ourselves that He had never let us down before. Our lives had already included many periods of waiting: the almost four years of infertility before we were able to have our second son and a two-year green card application process. Out of those waiting seasons we were able to declare to each other that He has never let us down.

Gaps, similar to waiting periods, are those parts of a story that no one knows except you and God. I don't know if you've ever thought of the Bible in this light, but there are many gaps in it. I sometimes wonder about Moses's 40 years with the sheep. What was this man—raised in the extravagant luxury of Pharaoh's palace—thinking about in that season of his life? Or, what about Jesus Himself? The Bible recounts very few details of His early life, apart from some smaller incidents that took place in His youth. We are left to wonder about the remaining 30 years prior to the wedding in Cana. What were Simeon and Anna doing for all those years before Jesus showed up (see Luke 2:25-38)? How were they living their lives? How did they stay in touch with their God? What encouraged them to continue believing and hoping for the coming of their Messiah? I can only imagine what their gaps and waits were like. Unlike theirs, mine were not 30 or 40 years in duration. In fact, it actually feels as though what was prophesied over me came to pass: "This is going to be a bump in the road." It was a deep bump, but it didn't last too long.

What do we do in the midst of our gaps and waits? The good news is, when life has you traveling and you don't know where you're going, He does. That is when we push aside what we don't understand and allow the journey to take place. In the early days of 2008, I began a journey that changed me. And crazy though it is, although I would rather have not walked through it, I also wouldn't swap the experience. Journeys like mine are the "walking the walk" seasons. It's in those moments that talking the talk just won't cut it. And it's also in those moments that we begin to ask ourselves where we get the courage to walk the walk.

The truth is that we can't walk alone. I love the revelation that you only need the fruits of the Spirit when living in community. If you live in a cave, you can get by without them. You may have some issues with God, but your need for the fruit of the Spirit only really comes to the forefront when you live in community. Not only that, but when crises come, it is those very fruits of the Spirit released to you from the community that help sustain you.

We weren't meant to walk this life alone: we were meant to journey in community. In fact, the purpose of heaven's government is to create society and family. God the Father, God the Son, and God the Holy Spirit were present in heaven before the world was created. It was and is the most perfect society that has ever been: the original government of heaven and earth. From that place of relationship, the Trinity had a vision and they created. And that's what government is meant to be. It's meant to be about relationships. It's meant to be about a society. The trouble is, here on earth, we end up defining government as management and maintenance instead of relationship, creativity, and vision. We are meant to live with people around us who feed us out of their relationships, out of the glory that they have from heaven. That is what Jesus's prayer in John 17:5 means: *"Now, Father, glorify Me together with Yourself, with the glory which I had with You before the world was."* He asked for this so that He could give it to us; that the world would know how we are meant to live life—in relationships of love, honor, and loyalty.

During my journey, I had my wife and my two wonderful sons by my side, but I, the guy who doesn't receive help very easily, had to learn how to receive. The Bethel team, the most amazing team on the planet, surrounded me. My best friend, Craig, who lives in San Diego, flew 750 miles to Redding for both the day of my diagnosis and surgery. Kris Vallotton, who doesn't like hospitals, also came to the doctor with me to hear the results of my tests, believing and hoping it would be good news. These relationships are priceless at such times. To have this kind of strength added to you is absolutely invaluable.

My doctor knew that there were two men in my life who would walk into a doctor's office to sit by me while I received my diagnosis. That was a testimony of love, relationship, and brotherly affection that the world needs to see. We were not meant to walk this life alone. But the truth is, you have to invest in your relationships before the crisis comes. Otherwise, there may not be relationships to experience when you need them most.

The courage for the journey comes from relationships, from having people that can speak into your life. And it comes from doing the things that you know to do. Have I put everything I've written into practice? No. Do I understand all there is to understand about this life, this journey, and how best to walk it out? No. But I had an aggressive cancer and I had to do some things aggressively. There were some things that my wife and I knew to do: take communion as often as we could, walk together, and read Dodie Osteen's book, *Healed of Cancer*. It's a tiny little book with 40 healing verses. Sue and I walked around the trails near our house, reading to each other, praying the verses over each other. We prayed them before we went to bed and prayed them when we got up in the morning. We did the things that we knew to do, and we did them as aggressively as we could. We got as much prayer as we could. I even had the entire first-year class of the School of Supernatural Ministry at Bethel pray for me.

On this journey, I was also given permission to not know, or even expect to know, all of the answers. I love the book written by 13th-century mystics, *The Cloud of Unknowing*. The basic message of the book is that we should put the things that we do not understand in an imaginary cloud to the left or right of our view of God. In this way, none of our questions or doubts obscures our view of God. That is 700-year-old wisdom, yet it stands the test of time. I have seen the importance of this truth played out as I have watched men and women stand in the midst of things that they do not understand, yet refuse to allow the pains and mysteries of life—which they do not have an answer for—to get in the way of their belief in the goodness of God.

In the gaps, waits, and journeys of life, especially the traumatic and tragic ones, there will likely be many things that we do not understand. Yet we can navigate wisely by choosing not to walk alone, by doing all we know to do, and by allowing ourselves to not have all the answers. We have been given permission to live with mystery and to know that faithfulness is always rewarded even if we do not reach what we believed was our destination. After all, the father of our faith, Abraham, was given his title as a result of the journey he took rather than his arrival at a destination.

Chapter 4

A Week of Kisses

Immediately after my first blood test result in January 2008, I had an extraordinary week. As the week progressed, I heard the Lord speak to me through people and circumstances, and I felt that He said, "I'll kiss you every day if you let Me." I knew, because of the context, that what He meant was, "I'll show you something every day if you let Me open your eyes to see in the midst of this journey and look above the circumstances. I will show you in ways unique and personal to you."

Bill Johnson, in his book *Dreaming with God,* talks about unusual circumstances and unusual coincidences. The Lord taught me that language a while ago when I was in a healthy season of my life (for want of a better description). He taught me to recognize the unusual circumstances and the coincidences of life that have His undeniable hand on them. I learned it most one day in 2005 when Bill said to me, "Paul, you have an assignment to pray for people with Down's syndrome." Earlier that weekend at a conference, a blond-haired, two-year-old girl named Emma jumped into my lap and head-butted my belly more times than anyone else has ever head-butted my belly before. It was as if my stomach was a mini trampoline for her. In reality, I think little Emma, who had Down's syndrome, was trying to hug me. I prayed for her as she sat in my lap, and that night, for the first time in her life, she went to a diner and drank a milkshake through a straw. Up until that night she had to eat thickened fluids from a spoon, as she had no pharyngeal reflex. I am delighted to say that several years later, she still continues to eat and drink normally, and her social skills have also developed.

When Bill spoke those words to me, I accepted the assignment because I could see a pattern of events and coincidences that led up to that moment. Interestingly, the unusual circumstances and coincidences that marked this as my assignment continued after I accepted it. That same year I went to preach at a church on Father's Day. The pastor of the church said to me, in preparation for the sermon, "It's Father's Day, but we are not going to honor the fathers today. We are going to honor this seventy-five-year-old man who never became a father or a husband because he dedicated his life to raising his Down's syndrome sister who died last week." That is an unusual circumstance, so I shared the testimony of Emma and my assignment, and sure enough, that day in church, there was a little girl with Down's syndrome.

A few months later I was visiting a different church, and a mother gave an announcement at the beginning of the church service. She said, "My eight-year-old son has Down's syndrome. He's very cute, but he's developed this habit of looking up girls' skirts. It's very cute at eight, but at eighteen, it's going to be a problem. I need you, church, to stand with me." Another unusual circumstance!

When she finished her announcement, I called her son up to the front. His name was Joey, and he had both ADD and Down's syndrome. As he ran toward me to the front of the sanctuary, I said, "What do you want most, Joey?"

And he muttered, "To speak." He ran past me—as his mother was trying to explain his behavior to me—grabbed a microphone and spoke my name. I was later told that prior to that moment, Joey couldn't have done that.

Through Joey, Emma, and various other happenings, the Lord started teaching me to recognize unusual circumstances and coincidences in life. He is always speaking, but we are not always listening. This way of God speaking to me is, I now realize, a way He has talked to me in the past and since. Reminders, clues, kisses, heaven invading my world—not always mysteriously, but in language that I would increasingly learn—is hard to miss.

Among the many notes in the margin of my Bible is the following: "You don't need signs on a familiar route, but you do need signs on an unfamiliar one." At that point in my life, I was certainly on an unfamiliar route. I was in scary territory that I had watched other people walk through but had never been through myself.

So after many reminders of how to recognize God's voice in unusual circumstances, I was completely prepared for Him to shower me with a "week of kisses" in January 2008. I returned to work after my brief trip to Fresno and after having processed the results of my blood test. I went into work one day, and my co-worker, Nancy, told me that she had a dream about me. In the dream were pearls dropping from heaven. Now, we often talk about diamonds and gems in our culture, ones appearing miraculously. It would not have seemed far-fetched for Nancy to have a dream about diamonds or gems dropping from heaven. But instead, she had a dream about pearls. And I knew God was speaking to me.

The year before my birth, 1957, when I was newly in my mother's womb, my father preached a message at a local church. (For the British readers, he spoke in a place called Chadwell Heath, on the east side of London.) His message was called "The Twelve Gates are Twelve Pearls." Pearls are the product of pain that is submitted to the foot of the cross. It's my life message. I took the transcript of my father's sermon and published it as a chapter in my first book, *What on Earth is Glory?* When Nancy told me there were pearls dropping from heaven, and that I was about to create another pearl through the pain of the journey, I knew that her dream was for me.

The next day Steve, our CPA, also shared a dream he had about me. Steve told me how I was about to have authority in a particular area of my life, specifically authority over prostate cancer as well as cancer in general. The following morning I taught in a marketplace meeting. At the end of the meeting, a man I'd never met came up to me and told me that he didn't know whether I was going up a mountain, coming down a mountain, or standing on it, but there was a mountain and it would be part of my testimony. Each unique encounter provided me with a fresh reminder of God's nearness.

The following day, someone who was on a similar journey approached me out of the blue, and I knew God was speaking to me. In fact, He was speaking to me in my language, familiar language—divine coincidences and unusual circumstances. Here's my point: in that type of season, when it can feel that no one around you can quite understand what you are experiencing, there is One who knows. And He sends messages, if you are looking for them—sweet messages, good messages, messages from the heart of a good God, pearls dropping from heaven just for you and me.

Another kiss I experienced along the way was a particularly sweet one. My wife Sue and I had experienced four years of infertility between the births of our two sons. When our eldest son, James, was nearly four years old, we were at a large event called Spring Harvest that is held every Easter in England. Faith Forster was speaking one afternoon, and at the end of her message she gave a word of knowledge about infertility, which was the condition my wife was experiencing. A few of our friends gathered around us and we prayed for Sue. That same night, in the main session, we sang the song with the line, "Nothing is too difficult for Thee," knowing the truth of that statement in our hearts, if not our experiences. Two weeks after that, Sue found out she was pregnant.

Nearly 20 years later, we were living in a community where we have never—to my knowledge—sung that song. Crystal, who was at that time working in a medical office with my wife, stood behind her one day and began to sing over her. Through a simple song, she sparked a memory from 1987 that had a victory attached to it. "Nothing is too difficult for Thee. Nothing, nothing, absolutely nothing. Nothing is too difficult for Thee." That moment was a demonstration of the pure goodness of God. Crystal could have sung a dozen other songs, but she chose that one—the one song that touched a memory and reminded us of a moment when God came through for us.

I have come to realize that we sometimes attribute cancer to God. We so easily make this mistake simply because God is so good at working with difficult situations. He works so closely and so intricately in our lives that sometimes it can almost seem as though He sent the challenge that He is so tirelessly guiding us through. You see, He is the Master Craftsman. I once heard Bill Johnson quote a prophetic word he received: "God does not remove the scars from your life, but He works with them so closely that they resemble finely carved crystal." That's our God. We mistakenly attribute God with causing the negative, instead of realizing that when God sees the difficult situations, His goodness says, "I will restore, I will re-create, and I will work so closely with it that it will become beautiful, so absolutely beautiful once again."

One morning I woke suddenly at two o'clock and thoughts began to invade my head. To distract myself, I leaned over and grabbed my iPhone to see what e-mails had come through. Just as I did that, an e-mail came through from Harrogate, England, that read, "We just had a prayer meeting, Paul. We had two circles. The inner circle was for everyone who was sick. The outer circle consisted of the prayer team. And I stood in for you. And they prayed for you."

On the day I actually got my diagnosis, I had a guest staying in my house. He is the son of the woman, Faith Forster, who led the meeting in which my wife was healed of infertility. Not only that, but 27 years before, this man had been healed of cancer. And here he was, staying in my house the day I received an official diagnosis of cancer. It was simply another case of God telling me that He was with me on this journey.

Although He had only promised a week of kisses, these kisses continued throughout my journey: phone calls, e-mails from heroes whom I had never met, and even an e-mail from the granddaughter of one of my all-time heroes. They never stopped encouraging me, whether directly from God, other people, or through unusual circumstances. My week of kisses became months of kisses from a good, good God—for which I will always be grateful.

Chapter 5

Encouraged by Heaven

For several years I had listened to reports of people going on "adventures" to heaven. These journeys included incredible healings, extravagant trances, and experiences of the imagination. To be honest, I was a bit resistant to experiencing this for myself, thanks to my analytical mind getting in the way of such an encounter. I allowed myself to ask too many questions rather than embrace the adventure with a childlike spirit. I wanted to know how, in fact, one could get to heaven, and once there, how one would know it was a valid experience.

Thankfully, Beni Johnson and Judy Franklin have helped immensely with their book, *Experiencing the Heavenly Realm*. Here is a quick taste:

> I have had the privilege to teach on heavenly encounters and have had people share their experiences afterward. I taught on this at a workshop in one of the youth conferences that we were having at the church. When I was done teaching, I told the participants that we were going to soak in God's presence and that many of them in the room would have heavenly experiences. When we were finished, I asked them if any would like to share what happened to them. One youth raised his hand and told us that when he was three, his parents died and that

when he was soaking, he was taken up into
Heaven and he saw his mom and dad.[1]

The crisis of cancer caused me to throw caution
to the wind. I asked Judy if I could have a personal
appointment. It was a conference week at Bethel,
which is always a busy time, but Judy made time for
my analytical mind and me. So, on February 28th,
2008, I lay on my office floor and Judy sat in a chair,
and she began to take me on a trip to heaven. That
date is probably insignificant for most people (unless
it is a birthday or anniversary). For me, however,
it happened to be the 35th anniversary of both my
father's passing and of my personal commitment to
Jesus. Judy began our time by saying, "I was praying
about this trip to heaven last night. And the Lord told
me to ask you to do something that I haven't ever
asked anyone else to do. He told me to ask you to
imagine speaking to your father."

This was certainly an unusual circumstance that
was about to get more unusual. Let me explain my
experience to you. I began by visualizing a shadowy
Jesus and myself as a baby in His arms. He nuzzled
His face into my face. I asked Jesus to show me the
world from heaven, and I could see it spinning on its
axis. Judy then said that there are gardens to explore
in heaven, but as she said that I saw earth become
a large pearl. I also had a sense that there were 11
other entrance points to heaven and that they were

like planets. I passed through the pearlescent earth as though it were mist, and then there opened out in front of me a view of mountains, water, and reflections. I focused on the water and a massive waterfall, which I could ride down. I rode that waterfall down and down. I then heard Judy tell me to imagine speaking to my father.

I imagined my father standing in front of me, and I began to ask him some questions in my mind. In my encounter, I somehow knew that my father lives by a river and is friends with Earl Johnson, Bill's father. In my mind, I asked him why this was so, and he said it was because we are family. In that moment, Jesus told me my father had died too early, but that He used it for great good. I then began to talk to Jesus and asked Him about my illness. He said that the Lion of the Tribe of Judah had taken care of it. When I mentioned the word *cancer*, He said, "What cancer?"

At one point I saw the entrance to hell being reduced in size and I had a sense that Satan's access to use light for his purposes was being reduced. A bit later I saw myself as a young man, and Jesus had me climb up a mountain where there were wildcats. I played with them and even put my head in their mouths. I knew that what I fear would eventually become like a playmate.

In my mind, I somehow knew that I could travel however I liked in heaven, so I went under the sea into the belly of a whale. I also saw something flying and was told—because in heaven we are sometimes told things through a sense of all-knowing—it was an elder flying around the throne. But the throne was the size of a planet, and I felt in that moment that my vision of God and heaven was way too small. Suddenly, I was walking over the earth with Jesus, and He was telling me that the gift of faith is how you see. He said that you could walk on earth seeing it as substance, or choose for it to be like a vapor.

And then my journey was over—I knew something had changed. In my opinion, the test of any experience like that is whether it changed you and pointed you to Jesus. Honestly, if a heavenly or supernatural experience doesn't change you or point you to Jesus, I can't believe it's an authentic experience. God wouldn't create an experience that didn't bring transformation and draw you closer to Him.

Two days later, I was at home having a Sozo—an inner healing session—with Dawna and Steve De Silva. As we began, I asked Dawna to minister concerning lust and pornography, as I knew that both could be related to the type of illness that was in my body. These things were not an issue in my life, but I wanted to be sure that there wasn't anything hidden or unseen. I knew that I had seen more than I wanted to on the walls of prisoners' cells when I worked in the prison system. Dawna told me that she did not feel that this was a problem. She then told me that the night before she had been praying for me and went to heaven in preparation for my Sozo. While she was there, Jesus gave her a scroll. When she unrolled the scroll, there in the middle was a picture of the Lion of the Tribe of Judah.

"Does that mean something?" she asked. Did it ever! So I told her about the excursion into heaven I had a few days prior. She understandably got very excited.

Fortunately, Sue was away in Moravian Falls that weekend; otherwise, I might have been too embarrassed to follow through with Dawna's next thought. She said, "You've got to step through this line in your life. But, when you press through this line in your life, you have got to roar like the Lion of the Tribe of Judah."

In my front room? I thought. *What if people are watching?*

Despite my fears, Dawna and Steve had me roar. And I have to say that I did them proud with my roar. I had to find righteous anger somewhere within myself. Sometimes I think I'm just too nice. I almost have this the-devil-really-ought-to-get-saved kind of feeling. But then I remember that Jesus fashioned a whip—He created it and then went in and deliberately beat the butts of the guys in the temple. He knew exactly what He was doing. He didn't just pick something up in a wild rage and use it to destroy the moneylenders' tables. He *fashioned* a whip. This was a lesson that I needed to learn. I too had to find—maybe even fashion—righteous anger inside of myself. I had to roar like a lion. I had to get at this thing that was attacking me, this thing that was robbing me.

God had given my analytical mind the confirmation it needed. My question all along had been, "How do I know this is real?" The Lion of the Tribe of Judah took care of that. These kinds of experiences vary from sanctified imaginings all the way to full trances, like those described throughout Scripture. My only concern is that when I experience something like this, the Holy Spirit is the tour guide and the result brings me closer to Jesus.

Endnote

1. Judy Franklin and Beni Johnson, *Experiencing the Heavenly Realm* (Shippensburg, PA: Destiny Image, 2011), 212.

Chapter 6

Saved by a Dream

I have few dreams that I can actually remember. It is not that I don't often dream; I just haven't often awoken with an awareness of what I may have been dreaming about. I am, in fact, jealous (in a healthy way, of course) of those who remember their dreams, and especially those who are guided by dreams. It is probably true that I have received more from dreams others have had about me than I have from my personal dream life. What happened in October 2007 is the most significant example.

One Sunday morning at church, Beni Johnson approached me and told me that she had a dream that involved me. It seemed, at first, that the dream was probably about Bethel, and I was just in it. But when she told me the dream, I somehow knew that there was something in it for me. Here is the dream, as given to me by Beni:

> I was walking with Paul toward a land split. Two pieces of land separated by a waterway. On the other side of the waterway was a city, which people entered through a gate. It looked like something in Israel when you go into the Old City. There was a sense that we were on one side and our staff and church family were all on the gate side. They had all gotten across the water.
>
> As we got to the water to cross over, there was no bridge. It seemed you had to jump. I knew

I could not make it across, so I was looking for the narrowest place. Paul, however, ran and jumped over. I thought he would make it because I had seen him do it before. But right as he jumped, we both knew that he wouldn't make it. So he did a side dive into the water. It was a very aggressive move. He dove sideways and twisted his body at the same time. I watched him go into the water and he didn't come up. I yelled to the other side for help; I'm not a good swimmer. Two people came running. The first person was Paul and the second person was a girl that owns a toy store in Redding. Yes, it was Paul that dove into the water.

Paul dove in first and then this gal. They both had no success. We thought Paul had drowned. I had crossed the water by then and was actually in the water. We were very upset and didn't know what to do. I took one last look at the water and saw bubbles come up: first one, then two, and then three bubbles. I yelled and said, "He's right there!" The two divers didn't see the bubbles, so I swam over and showed them. "Right here," I said. Paul dove into the water, swam down, and began coming up. Although I couldn't see him, I felt him coming up with the person drowned. I groaned inside of me to where it felt like travail. My travail was connected to Paul being able to come up.

When he came up out of the water, Paul the diver had a young man. He wasn't dead, but still alive and conscious. I looked at him and said, "I saw the bubbles."

He said to me, "You saw the bubbles." This young man was the young man who plays the star role in *Harry Potter*.

When I first heard this dream, I put a call out to any dream interpreters to give me their interpretation. That call led me into a relationship with a very fine young man, who would not only offer me an incredible interpretation, but also would, on occasion, travel with me and become like a spiritual son. Here is his interpretation:

Well, I feel that this is what the dream means in full. First of all, Beni had the dream, and that this dream would be in the category of an Intercession Dream makes sense since she's a hardcore intercessor. This category falls into the type of dreams that are in the five percent or less category, when dreams are about other people or things than the person dreaming. I'll break it down for you, then put it back together again.

First of all, Beni running alongside of you would be a picture of the intercessors, those who have been lifting you up in prayer and coming alongside the apostolic covering of Bethel Church in your life. Secondly, when you mentioned Beni couldn't make the jump, but you tried to, here's what I feel that means: the intercessors could only go so far alongside you. There were certain things that you had to battle one-on-one, you against your soul, to overcome the opposition against your life. As for halfway there, realizing you couldn't make it, that is a picture of your struggle in that season. The other side was the goal, the finish line to your healing. The river was the mysterious realm in between you and your goal, which was to get completely healed.

Jumping in after yourself to save yourself was the first key to your victory. Before you could overcome this opposition, the enemy—as you mentioned it in your sermon—you had to be fully secure in your confidence and focused on the light of the Lord's goodness. No grey zones, but fully in the light.

Finally, you rescuing the character of Harry Potter: I believe this is one of the main keys to interpreting this dream. I feel what this means is that through your victory over cancer, you will have the weapon—the "Goliath's sword" so to speak—around your waist to annihilate the spirit of death haunting those in the world who are going through what you went through. In this dream, God has transferred to you an anointing, signaling the release of captives and prisoners from this disease. Snatching sheep and goat alike, believer and non-believer, from the jaws of hell and bringing them into the fullness to which they were created. Your testimony of the Lord's goodness in your life will free many prisoners and captives who are bound by the occult and witchcraft. The child in them will truly be set free to be childlike and joyful in the Lord, and the false anointing of power will be revealed for what it truly is: false.

So to put the interpretation in one or two sentences, the dream, I feel, means this: you went through a difficult season, where there were things you had to face personally. But you strengthened yourself in the Lord, and as a result of your personal triumph, there will be corporate breakthrough—particularly for those bound by cancer and demonic oppression and disease, snatching them from the jaws of death and bringing them into the knowledge of God's glory and goodness.

I believe that the last part of that dream, involving the character that plays Harry Potter, represents a principality. We are living in a season when the light is going to shine on principalities. And when the light shines on them, they will be revealed for exactly what they are. One such principality that will be revealed is that which is stopping the world from knowing and believing that God is good.

The other significant aspect of the dream is that it activated my subconscious to save my own life. I was in the hospital over Easter weekend for my surgery, and during that time I nearly died. The last thing I remember on Friday afternoon, after my surgery, was a conversation with Kris Vallotton, who was visiting me. We talked briefly—for some strange reason— about Mordecai. The next thing I knew, I was being woken up with the results of a cardiac enzyme test, which, being a nurse, I knew meant that they suspected I had cardiac problems. I hadn't even been aware of my blood being taken. I cannot imagine how scared Sue must have been during those hours when I was oblivious to everything.

I lay in bed, drifting in and out of sleep, when I was awoken by the alarm on my blood pressure monitor indicating that my mean arterial pressure was dangerously low. At 2:27 a.m., Saturday morning, after I had experienced 12 hours of dangerously low blood pressure, it occurred to me that there didn't seem to be anybody around that was going to solve this problem. The blood pressure machine was going off every seven minutes, and my blood pressure kept dropping. Every once in a while, it would creep up a little bit, and then it would drop again.

As I lay in bed at 2:27 a.m., I said, "God, You need to give me wisdom for this." And He gave me wisdom. He reminded me that my kidneys control my blood pressure, to some extent, and that somehow, the catheter was affecting them. In a matter of 15 minutes, I got my blood pressure from 79 over 49 to 125 over 80. I won't go into the details, but my catheter wasn't draining. Once I had called the nurses and convinced them to check my catheter, it began to drain properly, and my blood pressure returned to normal. God gave me wisdom in the middle of the night. I believe that dream, the dream that activated my subconscious to fight for myself, actually saved my life. That's how good He is. Psalm 75:1 says, *"How we thank You, Lord. Your mighty miracles give proof that You care"* (TLB). I love that.

The Bible has so many examples of dreams and dream interpretations that it is, without doubt, foolish to ignore them. It reminds me of something Bill Johnson says about angels—we should not worship them, but it is foolish to ignore them. Dreams seem similar to me. It is unwise to make them our only guides, but it is equally unwise to ignore them. Imagine where Egypt and Pharaoh would have ended up had Pharaoh not dreamed and had Joseph not interpreted the dream.

Beni's dream somehow planted a thought in my soul, which I retrieved in the middle of the night while lying in the hospital. We do not have all of the answers and we do not know or understand everything that is going on in our lives. As you may well remember, Psalm 16 says that our mind instructs us in the night season. Semi-consciousness is definitely a night season, one during which my soul or spirit was prompted to awake and ask questions. This is most certainly an example of how God prepares us, even in unusual ways. As I reflect on that dream and how I felt when Beni first shared it with me, I recall that my spirit was stirred. Sometimes I can pass things by, but I am learning more and more to pay attention to His prompting.

One of my sons' favorite comedians uses the phrase, "Get their attention." I often feel that God is doing that to me. Sometimes it seems as if He is not even talking, but I think, more than likely, I am not listening, nor am I aware of the way in which He is speaking. This summer alone, I had three experiences in which I know God was speaking to me, not about anything directional or even a warning, but simply to get my attention. The first was on the day my first book was published. I sat in my office with a revivalist from Romania who had known my wife's grandfather—the same grandfather who gave me some key advice just after I first heard my call to ministry. That advice took me on a journey through nursing and prison management and equipped me for the role I fulfill today, a role far removed from anything I imagined when I first heard that call to ministry. Because of his advice, I was now sitting in my office with his old friend. God wanted to get my attention, perhaps for no other reason than to make sure I was listening.

The second instance took place in July, when I unexpectedly met the man who trained the man who introduced Sozo (inner healing) to Bethel. It is because of the inner healing ministry that Sue and I were even introduced to Bethel, and then dared to venture from the UK to California. Again, God was telling me to pay attention.

Finally, less than a month later, I had the privilege of sitting under Reinhard Bonnke in Chicago at the Jesus Culture Awakening conference. That moment served as a reminder for me. I was meant to hear Reinhard speak in the UK in 1989. I am convinced that if I had gone to hear him speak, as I was supposed to, then I may have prematurely pursued a journey away from prison management. These three events may not seem significant at one level, but they got my attention. In the same way, Beni's dream got the attention of my subconscious. I don't fully understand it, but I will be forever grateful that He bothers to get our attention, especially when we think He isn't even talking.

Chapter 7

A First-Class Healing

"Surgery is not a second-class healing." These simple words helped to begin a new leg of my life journey and introduce me to new friends and opportunities. I had not said them before in a sermon, but my journey through cancer had created an awareness of the need to say it publicly. Although I had laid down my nursing career nearly 30 years before, saying it enabled my return into the healthcare arena, which, to be honest, is a first love of my working life. I have had the greatest respect for the medical profession all of my life. I have worked alongside some of the finest men and women in the world of medicine and, in recent years, experienced first-hand what skill, power, and care they hold in their hands. What I had not realized was that in a culture of the supernatural, these professionals can, at times, feel second-class.

This second-class feeling, I have found, is not uncommon for Christians in careers outside of the Church. This is not the case, however, for some farmers I recently met in South Africa. These men raise cattle, and they really love their meat. It is they who taught me the "sanctity" of the *braai* (South African barbeque). As they filled the *braai* with red meat of all kinds, they humorously—with a degree of passion—told me that around them, chicken is considered a vegetable. As I spent time with them, I realized that their provision of meat is never considered a second-class ministry. After all, if quail could be provided

96

supernaturally or fish multiplied, then it could be considered that farming is a second-class provision of food. But that thought never enters their heads. These men are proud to be carrying on the tradition, begun in Genesis, of subduing and harvesting this planet for the benefit of mankind.

Not so with my journey through cancer, which raised questions and, at times, accusations and inferences that getting well through surgery or medicine is a second-class healing. On my journey, I met face-to-face, up close and personal, the challenge of my enemy, cancer. Diagnostic facts, statistics, and options were thrown at me, but this time not as a pastor, friend of a patient, or nurse, but as a newly diagnosed cancer patient who lives in the supernatural community of Bethel Church. Sue and I have been around cancer and sickness all of our lives, and we have talked many times about what we would do in the face of such trials. Our hearts have been broken repeatedly as we watched loved ones suffer with disease. But perhaps a greater pain has been when we have seen some refuse treatment in the name of faith and subsequently lose their lives. This does not deny that some have a clear word from the Lord to stand solely on their faith—people who I have the greatest respect and admiration for.

This chapter is not easy to write as I realize with every sentence that I may be accused of lacking faith.

But that, I can assure you, is not the case. If you need healing, and the healing comes by prayer alone, then that is wonderful! But if it doesn't come by prayer alone, and if we don't accept doctors as being ministers of healing, then we may make a very serious and life-threatening mistake. Apart from some extreme sects, I have never yet heard of anyone refusing an appendectomy in the name of faith. But I *have* heard of many who refuse treatment for treatable forms of cancer. I do know that sometimes chemotherapy and radiotherapy can be brutal, and I am not without concerns about that, but I will continue to look doctors in the eye and tell them that their ability to bring health does not qualify as a second-class healing.

As I have written in my book, *What on Earth is Glory?*, the definition that we place on glory will determine where we expect to encounter it. We are made in the image of God, who is Healer. Healing is not merely something He does; it is His identity. It is not, therefore, surprising that in His image we would heal, both through prayer and through mastering knowledge of the body that God created. To relegate medicine as inferior to supernatural healing will prevent us from seeing the glory that healthcare professionals carry, and it will deny them the awareness of the power of their ministry.

Of course, for most of us, prayer would be our first option. Within an hour of my diagnosis, I was surrounded by 600 of our School of Ministry students as they prayed for my healing. I would receive prayer from the Sunday school class of five-year-olds and welcome their prophetic declarations as well as the paintings from several of my colleagues' children. I would attend our Healing Rooms and—somewhat proudly—complete the section asking where I heard about the Healing Rooms with the statement that I started them!

I did not see the miracle I had hoped for. However, I became increasingly aware that some who live in a supernatural culture interpret the doctor's diagnosis as a curse. We need to be very careful that we do not view our doctors and healthcare providers as liars or as agents of the devil—our enemy and source of disease—although they are required to speak of what may appear negative. Doctors are trained to deliver a diagnosis, which is distinctly different from speaking a curse. The report of the Lord is, of course, that He heals, and we are to embrace this report. But we also must recognize that doctors daily experience the painful journeys traveled by their patients. We hopefully only rarely find ourselves exposed to the burden of a negative diagnosis, but for doctors and nurses, this represents their daily lives.

Now, nearly four years cancer free, as I visit my doctor, he talks to me of how rare appointments like mine are. We chat about cameras and my medical friends in the Dakotas, who are seeing miracles in their hospital on a regular basis. On one of my visits, not wanting to be a burden, I sent a message to the doctor that I didn't need to see him if he was too busy. When he finally got to my exam room, he was eager to tell me that he would not want to miss out on even 15 minutes with one of his successes! The truth is, the majority of his—and thousands of other healthcare professionals'—days are filled with bad news and sadness. To maintain a healthy outlook within these circumstances is a daily challenge made unbearably worse if their career is deemed second-class or their words considered a curse.

I was asked, on one occasion, to be father to a young woman who was given a terrible diagnosis. Very early one Saturday morning, as I sat by her bed with her husband, I watched the agonized look on the cancer specialist's face as he conveyed the worst of news. I was there to ask the questions that shock and pain often prevent us from being able to ask at such times. Little did I know that I would soon need my friends to sit with me in a similar exam room for the very same reason. One thing I know about that day, however, is that although the words of the diagnosis were devastating, they were not delivered as a curse. They were a diagnosis given by a man trained to know what he is talking about and what options remain for his patients. This particular oncologist is a wonderful and skillful Catholic believer, and he knew that a miracle was the only answer for this young woman. His work daily exposes him to tragedy, and he carries faith and the compassion of Jesus with him. He sees victories and losses. Yet, like many healthcare professionals, he has dedicated his life to heal and relieve the suffering caused by the real curse of disease.

My first career was as a nurse in one of the world's finest teaching hospitals. I have been privileged to stand in operating theaters (ORs) and see the incredible skill of a surgeon's hands. I have been the scrub nurse and, on one occasion, the surgeon's assistant. I am neither an expert nor a doctor, but I do know about the course that cancer takes and the trauma of treatment that can often cause symptoms that appear worse than the disease itself.

Whether thanks to my experience with healthcare, my faith in God, or simply the grace of the One who stood beside me, I chose to approach my situation by marrying the medical advice given me with the supernatural. I was given a diagnosis and advised by my doctor that immediate surgery was the best option. Armed with that information, I asked when the earliest appointment for surgery would be. As it was nearly four weeks away, I then asked if I could have a second biopsy as near to the surgery as possible. "I plan to receive prayer for healing," I told the doctor. "We have seen many healed of cancer and other diseases." I am pretty sure that he thought I was crazy to ask for a second biopsy, as they really are not very pleasant. But he honored my faith and my request. I did as I had planned, and when a second biopsy confirmed the continued presence of cancer, I proceeded to have the surgery.

It really is very important to say that the discovery of my cancer was, in and of itself, a miracle. The cancer was an aggressive one and my doctor told me after my surgery that he thought it was only a matter of days or weeks before it would have gone outside of my prostate, which would have been a critical and life-threatening development. Although I was not healed without surgery, I have experienced a couple of miracles since. They were continued kisses from heaven to tell me that, although healing didn't come the way I hoped it would, He is capable of working things out naturally or supernaturally.

The first of these miracles happened a month after my surgery, while I was facilitating a Strategic Planning Workshop. My scar from surgery is in the middle of my abdomen. At the time, while I had no pain near the scar, my groin was in agonizing pain. I think it was where the surgeon had placed the retractor during surgery, and potentially tore my groin muscle. I could walk, but I couldn't stand for more than 15 or 20 minutes without pain. The day of the workshop, I found myself at the beginning of a 12-hour day, knowing that for eight of those hours I would be on my feet. As I walked into the room at the start of the workshop, I immediately felt the presence of God. I decided to ask everyone in the room who was sick to stand up. Three-quarters of the room stood up, and I began to pray for them. As I was praying for one gentleman, I felt him start to fall under the Spirit, and, as I was about to catch him, I remembered that I was not supposed to lift any weight. So I moved my hand back, and the poor guy hit the deck! It was a case of him or me. After I had finished praying for 27 different people, my groin pain left. Nobody prayed for me. The pain simply left because of His presence, and it never returned.

A little while later, I was aware that my scar was not healing very well. It was extremely lumpy and uneven, and the doctor told me I needed to get a special cream. Sue and I were watching a revival conference on TV one night, when a word of knowledge was given for people with scars. In that moment, Sue leaned over and prayed that my scar would go, believing that the whole scar would disappear. She has great faith, my wife! She finished praying and I didn't think anymore about it. The next day came and went, and that evening I went to put some cream on my scar. To my surprise, the scar was completely smooth and has been ever since. These are kisses from a very good God!

My dream, one that I am honored to experience today, is of doctors and healthcare professionals who have married their training with the supernatural power of God. They do all that they know to do, and when they have opportunity, they pray. And as they have always done, they are seeing miracles. At a recent gathering of healthcare professionals, two doctor friends of mine shared testimonies of miraculous healings in their practices that occurred both with and without treatment. They added that my simple statement, that healing brought about through surgery and medicine is not second-class, changed the way they practice and view their careers. It was a humbling and encouraging moment as I realized that the healthcare career I left nearly 30 years before is still a part of my life.

One of those same doctors told the story of how he and an intern from Bethel's School of Supernatural Ministry prayed every day for his patients. As a result of this, they saw and documented an average reduction of length of hospital stay by one day per patient. They didn't see the hospital empty out, but they saw wellness come to the patients and the speed of recovery increase. That is a miracle. Whether healing comes instantaneously or whether it comes through process and modern medicine, the goal, may I remind you, is to get well.

Chapter 8

He Really Is Good

This chapter is the very thesis of this book and of my journey. God really is good! And no, He is not relatively good compared to something else. He is the standard by which all other goodness should and will be compared. All of us at Bethel Church in Redding, and those who experience Bill Johnson's preaching and ministry, are indebted to the manner in which he has refreshed this timeless truth and created a culture that embraces the goodness of God as if it were a brand new revelation.

Cancer had the audacity to visit while I was living in a culture where we openly declare the goodness of God. In day-to-day life, the word *good* is often used in comparison to some other experience. This is a misuse of the biblical understanding of the word. In the book of Genesis, we see that God created all things, and after the creation of every one of them "He saw that it was good" (see Gen. 1:10,12,18,21,25,31). I want to remind you that this statement of goodness included you and me. Maybe I should repeat that. God declared that His creation was good, and that included us.

After reading about how all things were created, we then read of man eating of the fruit of the tree of the knowledge of good and evil (see Gen. 3). There are various messages one could take from the trees in the garden, but I want to focus on just one aspect of these trees. Before Adam and Eve ate of this tree, they only had eyes to see the standard of goodness. After they ate the fruit of the tree, however, they entered a world of comparison between good and evil. From that moment in time, the lines began to blur, and the perspective of the viewer began to alter the concept of what is and isn't good or evil. Man began life made in His image, but the process of the fall accelerated to a perpetual state of falling, that is until Jesus came and, by His death and resurrection, returned to us the mind of Christ. He restored to us the capacity to know His goodness, not by comparison, but by revelation.

The kisses, the circumstances, and the things God showed me, said to me, and did for me all revealed that He is outrageously good. The first Adam saw God and the goodness of creation. The second Adam, Jesus, saw again the inherent goodness in mankind and came to shine a light that would reveal our full potential—a potential that would cause Him to die for us and judge for us.

There are two Bible references that are fairly well known, not for their true meaning, but almost entirely for a half-truth for which they have long been misinterpreted. Both references are ultimately related to the goodness of God. The first is recorded in Luke 15, the well-known story of the prodigal son. The word *prodigal* only appears in one verse and is really just a way of describing one of the main characters in the story. Bibles title that passage as the story of "The Prodigal Son," when it really should be famous for being the story of the extravagantly loving father! The father was extravagant when he gave the inheritance at the son's request, extravagant as he watched and waited for his son's return, extravagant when he ran to greet his son, when he fell on his son's neck, put a ring on his finger, robe on his back, and shoes on his feet, and extravagant when he ordered the roasting of the fatted calf. Who knows? Perhaps he constantly kept a fatted calf ready for that long-awaited moment! The father was also extravagant when he told the upset elder brother, *"All that is mine is yours"* (Luke 15:31). How few people, both outside and within the Church, really know this aspect of God—a loving, good God who restores all things to the original created order.

The second biblical reference that has been taken out of context is that of judgment day. A movie of that same name has brought an increased awareness to the world of an impending day of judgment, a day when many expect to be harshly judged for their choices while on earth. It is true that there will be a judgment day, but the full truth is that the heart of God is to judge for us, not against us. There is much confusion because, in many Bibles, the book of Revelation has a subheading titled "Judgment Day" (see Rev. 20:11-15). However, that phrase doesn't appear in the text itself. The text explains that God will send the Deliverer to judge for us—"us" being all of those whose names are in the Book of Life. It may be that all of our names began in the Book and then some got blotted out, or that the Book of Life starts with blank pages and gradually has names written in it. The former concept doesn't remove the need for us to have a relationship with God, but it does reveal God's heart that all of our names be in the Book of Life. Even throughout the book of Judges, God sent each individual judge to deliver the people to Him, not to condemn them. Surely He will be the best Judge we could hope for.

An incorrect view of God and the religious practices that stem from that have surrounded so much of our culture and left many believing that God would send cancer to teach us a lesson. Our God already sent a Teacher—His name is Jesus. Cancer didn't come to teach us a lesson; God sent Jesus to teach cancer a lesson! He came to reveal the Father. He is the Judgment and the Good Shepherd. He made a way where there is no way. His life, death, and resurrection are the manifestation of an outrageously good and loving God who was willing to endure separation from His Son in order to get His kids back! He is an extravagant Father while He waits; He will one day welcome us home with identity, authority, and sonship; and we will all get to celebrate and be celebrated with a lavish feast!

Cancer is a principality. A simple definition of a *principality* is "an area or aspect of life on earth that is dominated by darkness and the rulers of darkness." Paul writes that it has its roots in our minds: *"We are destroying speculations and every lofty thing raised up against the knowledge of God, and we are taking every thought captive to the obedience of Christ"* (2 Cor. 10:5). The principality of cancer isolates people, brings fear into their lives, and ultimately robs them of life before and after death, if it is allowed to. It will introduce a new language into people's lives, take them out of the norm, rob them of joy, and stop them from living. It is a principality that stands in direct opposition to the goodness of God.

I believe that there are principalities that will be undone simply when the world finds out how good God is. The world has been exposed to the wrong view of our God, and it is our responsibility to correct it. It is our responsibility to bring about a cultural transformation. *Culture* is the collection of beliefs, traditions, and customs held by a group of people and is their way of coping with the world. That culture is then passed from generation to generation through education and learning. When we pass along an understanding of His goodness, however, we will see the culture transformed and principalities undone. The world will know truth, and they will flock to worship a God they have been held back from. You have insurance policies that don't pay out if there's an "act of God." Somehow, we've attributed to Him atrocities that do not belong to Him. A revelation of His goodness will change all of that.

The good news is that it is possible to walk through cancer and still access the goodness of God. This experience, of the three or four darkest months of my life, revealed all the more that He is absolutely and utterly good. I know there are people who need to know the truth of His goodness because of the situations or challenges they are facing. In fact, if you are one of those people, I want to encourage you that it may be in the midst of such circumstances that the revelation of His goodness will be richest. The goodness of God is a light that shines on a principality and starts to break it into pieces.

Kris Vallotton preached an amazing message on this very topic right while I was in the midst of learning this valuable lesson. He said, "A powerless life is a life caused by forgetting who you are, who He is, and His plan for your life." So I began to work on these things. I felt at times like everything I had believed and even preached for the past five years of my life was standing up and looking me in the face and saying, "Do you still believe that now?"

In one of my teachings, I unwrap the passage in Exodus that details Moses's journeys up the mountain to meet with God (see Ex. 34:29-35). And I ask my audience and myself, "What was it that caused

Moses's face to shine?" I read that it is not the first, or even the second, but the third trip down the mountain when Moses's face begins to shine. For 40 days, Moses heard the voice of God about the building of the tabernacle, and he received the tablets that were carved by God's hand and written with His finger. However, it wasn't his proximity to God's presence or even the consuming fire that caused his face to shine. It was on the third trip up the mountain that God revealed to Moses how good He was. It was His goodness that made the face of Moses shine. I adamantly believe that God's goodness changed Moses's complexion; yet, in the midst of fighting cancer, it felt like that message was standing up and looking me in the face, saying, "Will you still say that I am good?" *Yes, I will,* I thought. *You're still good.* To daily remind myself of that truth, every e-mail I sent during that season was signed, "He's still good."

One day in particular I began to wonder if I could still hear the voice of God. I asked myself, "Do I hear You anymore, God, in the middle of all this?" That same day, a team happened to be visiting Bethel from Southern California. I only had five minutes to spend with them as I had a scheduled doctor's appointment that day. In those five minutes, I gave them a prophetic word about paradigm shifts and moving from camel farming to ship building. The team immediately responded that they had preached about that same thing a few days before. It was so encouraging to know that I was still hearing God in the midst of my crisis.

However, I also began to realize that the enemy was trying to attach my identity to my crisis. But then I read in Isaiah 43:1, *"Do not fear, for I have redeemed you; I have called you by name; you are Mine!"* From there, Isaiah goes on to say that we may go through storms, floods, and fires, but those circumstances will not change the truth of the preceding verse. He has called you by name, and He will be with you in the storm, the fire, the river, the earthquake, and beyond. Our identity is not in the crisis. I was not named by my crisis, but by who I am in Him.

The apostle Paul reveals how crises can enhance our knowledge of God. During this season, I started to read parts of Paul's letters chronologically; and as I read Paul's account of being beaten, shipwrecked, and imprisoned, I realized that the following passage from Romans was written after those experiences:

> *For I am convinced that neither death, nor life, nor angels, nor principalities, nor things present, nor things to come, nor powers, nor height, nor depth, nor any other created thing, will be able to separate us from the love of God, which is in Christ Jesus our Lord* (Romans 8:38-39).

This verse is not mere theology. It is theology in action, which very well may be a great definition of *kingdom.*

If one man knew all of the things that could possibly separate a person from feeling the love of God, it was the apostle Paul; yet he was still able to write that nothing can truly separate us from His love. It's because life isn't a theology; it's a biography. The trouble is, we turn Paul's writing into theology, and some forget that his biography is theology in action. He lived it. It happened to him. He walked through it. His was a real life in relationship with a real God. A real life in relationship with a real God who is so utterly good, that He brought Paul through every one of those tests and trials and shipwrecks and disasters, and at the end of it, Paul could still write, *"For I am convinced that neither death, nor life...will be able to separate us from the love of God...."*

My goal is simply to encourage you. No matter what you are going through, He is good, and He wants you to know that. His goodness may be revealed in many diverse ways, but your circumstances do not determine His goodness. All of us want to see our cultures transformed, and I believe that a key to cultural transformation is to manifest, demonstrate, and tell the world that no matter what we're walking through, no matter what is happening to us, He is good.

Chapter 9

Shine the
Light

Jesus says of Himself that He is the Light of the world. Even though I knew He said this, I was surprised to read in John 9:5 that He said, *"While I am in the world, I am the Light of the world."* This put a fresh emphasis on Matthew 5:14, in which Jesus says that *we* are the light of the world. Knowing this suddenly puts our responsibility into perspective. We are meant to be light to this world.

If principalities are spiritual places ruled by darkness, then light must be the answer to overcoming principalities. As I have already said, principalities, at least in part, exist in the mind. We are called to be light, light that demolishes principalities and raises the standard of His goodness. It is the very core of cultural transformation. Psalm 119:105 declares, *"Your word is a lamp to my feet and a light to my path."* The psalmist is saying that whatever it is that comes against us in life, we should be able to walk through it in such a way that we never lose sight of His goodness, simply because His light is shining through us and onto our path.

I am going to express a rather profound thought now, and you need to fasten your seatbelts for this: Darkness is dark; and light eradicates darkness. There are many thoughts that enter into the head of a person who suffers disease or crisis, especially if that person has an underlying, false belief that God sent it. If we believe that God sent our diseases, then we believe we are being punished, causing us to live in shame—hiding our experience in the dark and refusing to expose it to the light. But if light can shine on the false belief that God causes disease, then judgment will be released, the judgment that reveals His goodness. In this way, the tables will immediately be turned, no longer against you but against the author of darkness.

Judgment is light. Jesus brought this with Him when He came, but He left it with us. When we use the word *judgment* in relationship to God, we must see the truth: He desires to judge for us. In the same way, when we shine light, we release judgment, not against people but against darkness. Cancer brings its own darkness with it, and then, with the addition of false beliefs, the darkness can quickly grow darker. Perhaps that is what is meant by "deep darkness" in Isaiah 60:2: *"For behold, darkness will cover the earth and deep darkness the peoples."* Darkness can also be a place where we choose to leave good things and experiences. If we leave what is good in the darkness, there is no testimony to share with others. And, if there is no testimony, there is no prophecy of who Jesus is. And if there is no prophecy, there are people who are walking the same path in the darkness, who will not know that it's possible to access light in the middle of their journey.

Our job then is to shine the light of heaven directly at the darkness. I don't know the statistics, but I have a very strong conviction that more people recover from cancer than die from it. That news could considerably reduce that cancer-caused darkness. In fact, somebody said to me that he watched a TV program about people who live to be over 100 years old. One of the common denominators of all of those people was that they had beaten cancer at some stage in their lives.

Living and ministering at Bethel Church in Redding, I am part of an apostolic move of God and I oversee Global Legacy, Bethel's apostolic, relational network of revival leaders. In this environment we are learning that a significant characteristic of an apostolic, societal transforming movement is the stewardship of heaven's culture here on earth. Culture, rather than doctrine, has become a focus for us. That is not to say that what we believe isn't important, but it is second in line to creating a culture where our beliefs can grow to maturity rather than be squelched by the fires of academic arguments and disagreements.

Culture depicts two images for me. The first is of a petri dish, as in a science lab, where there is a medium in which a culture is encouraged to grow. The second image is of Spain, where, in order to avoid the heat of the noonday sun, the culture of a daily siesta has been established. The phrase "mad dogs and Englishmen go out in the noonday sun" was birthed in Spain. While taking a siesta to avoid the heat is an instinctive part of Spanish culture, visiting English men and women do not automatically have that cultural instinct.

These two pictures help me to interpret what it means to bring heaven's culture to earth. Much like the petri dish, our goal is to create a medium that allows the culture of heaven to grow. The origin of the medium will determine what actually grows. The origin of cancer is hell, and, not surprisingly, what grows in that medium looks, tastes, and feels like hell! Cancer, above all, provokes fear and provides a medium in which hopelessness and despair grow free. I understand that those of you who have battled cancer are probably thinking that the effects of cancer treatment are sometimes hellish as well and can feel worse than the disease itself. However, as I have already said in Chapter 7, those treatments are often heavenly revelations given to men and women to help destroy this disease, both medically and surgically, in the absence of a divine miracle. The culture created by cancer is one of an all-encompassing fear and hopelessness—something that affects the mind, body, and soul.

Throughout my years of nursing, and the various encounters I have had with cancer patients, I've observed that what is all-invading is the domination of the patient's and family's lives by the culture that comes with cancer. So much of what cancer brings is unavoidable. But I do not believe that it should be allowed to take over unchallenged. All of a sudden, routines are changed, diet and daily activities affected, language altered, and all because of the "c" word. Of course, this applies to most other diseases and personal crises, but cancer has cornered the market, it seems, in the area of a disease to be universally feared.

For this reason, we need a counterculture—and heaven provides it. Every hell-originated component of culture has a match from heaven, and not just a match, but a match winner. Fear is conquered by love, hopelessness by hope. The challenge throughout the journey of disease is allowing exposure to the medium in which heaven's culture grows and chokes out the life of hell. Praying that heaven's culture is revealed through many and diverse ways, including through friends, family, and even healthcare professionals, is valid. Our pursuit is that heavenly culture would become an instinctive part of our daily lives, just as the siesta is an instinctive part of a Spaniard's life.

Recently, a lady in the early days of her chemotherapy treatment visited my office. We had prayed three weeks prior that the culture of the kingdom would surround her. I was so happy to hear her report that the surgeon planning for her post-chemotherapy surgery had said that she might already be healed. The sound of the word "healed" was so encouraging to her; it's a kingdom word, used by a surgeon and spurred on by heaven. Healed is final: it's not remission, not living in fear of the disease returning. Needless to say, it encouraged her soul. That lady walked bravely through arduous treatment, regularly coming to me and others for prayer, and she has now been declared cancer free. It was as if, in her case, the diagnosis was a benchmark for a miracle, delivered by doctors with help from heaven.

Remember the image of the Spanish siesta, the culture that protects us from the fierce rays of earth's noonday sun? The culture of this world will tell us that God sent cancer to punish or discipline us. This message is not only wrong, but also terribly confusing, conflicting with the message of God's love and goodness that we all truly need to receive. God cannot send something to earth that He does not have. Figuratively speaking, the mindset that He does send disease will destroy us. It will burn us up if we let it, disintegrating our awareness of a good God and leaving us more and more in the hands of the culture of earth. Instead, we need to create a culture much like the siesta: providing rest and respite from the harsh effects of life on a fallen earth. Worship, soaking, fellowship, and God's presence are all helpful practices. My wife and I also chose to pursue life. Sue's repeated phrase was, "We have to live." In other words, we both knew that cancer would not become our environment.

Creating and living in such a culture will require some courage and, at times, the exercise of boundaries. You see, after a diagnosis has been given, out of the woodwork come many and various opinions for the patient to consider, from weird treatments to accusations that if we had eaten better we could have avoided the cancer. I know that there is an element of truth in these things: diet is a vital part of health. But in my case, however, someone actually sat down next to me and told me that my diet had caused my cancer. This person didn't know me, nor had she ever eaten a meal with me or observed my dietary habits. We all need helpful advice at such times, and it is out there, but practicing boundaries is also an important part of the journey. In this particular case, I was so grateful to have my wife coach me in my boundaries. And I knew that, while carefully monitoring my diet would be important, my diet was not the cause of my cancer!

I have already shared how my time as a nurse exposed me to disease and the resulting effects. However, what I have not shared much is that my exposure to cancer's culture was early on in life as I walked with my father through his own cancer journey. I remember days spent driving to the specialist, constantly changing routines, and, to be honest, few people stepping in with the weapons to combat that ugly culture. Watching him fight his battle with very little outside help has caused me to be drawn to those fighting a similar battle, but with one primary goal: changing the culture around them. It is, sadly, very likely that most of us will have the opportunity to walk with someone through cancer. However, we can consider it to be our opportunity to create a culture where healthy things are allowed to grow, and where those we walk with get to experience the siesta of heaven.

Hope grows in the wilderness. It rarely grows, nor does it need to, in the oasis of life. As Hosea puts it, God will *"make the valley of Achor* [trouble] *as a door of hope"* (Hos. 2:15). Cancer will try to shut the "door of hope" or, more likely, tell you that one does not exist. And somehow, the spirit of hopelessness will find a way in. A life of hopelessness brings premature death, even though the vital signs may still be present. Proverbs says, *"Hope deferred makes the heart sick"* (Prov. 13:12). Our heart does not become sick because we don't get what we hope for. It becomes sick when we stop hoping altogether. The culture of heaven will always bring hope. Never be afraid of false hope—hope in God can never be false.

As we battle the principality of disease, we must remember that it is simply darkness, and we are the light of the world. When a culture opposite to heaven's culture threatens to invade your world, remember to shine His light. Get prayer, worship, eat well, make sure you live in the light of His presence, and go to the doctor. Walk through all of the steps, but take some light, hope, joy, and love with you. They will be your best companions and guides.

Chapter 10

Family: God's Big Idea

On my return from the doctor's office after receiving my diagnosis, I stood in Bill Johnson's office, the senior leader of Bethel Church. For those of you who know him and the movement originating from his ministry, you may immediately think that his office is one of the best places to be on the whole planet after receiving bad news. I would agree with you. After my worst fears were realized earlier that day in the doctor's office, I sat in Bill's office and watched as my wife of 29 years became devastated by the news that her husband had cancer. I have come to realize that, many times, it is the spouse who bears the greater burden in these circumstances. They cannot afford the luxury of self-pity as the diagnosis propels them into a support role.

As we sat there, Bill asked me a defining question. One of Bill's greatest characteristics is that he draws truth by asking questions. This was not a moment for sympathy; this was a moment to find truth that would equip me for the fight. Few men I know can find the question at that poignant moment, when faced with someone else's pain. It is not that Bill is not a compassionate person—quite the contrary—but he has an ability to stay above circumstances and minister from heaven, as he did for me that day.

I remember, although somewhat dazed at the time, trying to process the news while looking across the room at Bill. He asked me, "What do you think the fight is about, Paul?" I am certain that was not what I expected to have anyone ask, but it was Bill's way of shining light. Even after the question had been delivered, I had no idea how powerful the subsequent answer would be from that moment, and for weeks and even years to come.

In response, I looked down at my lap and pondered. Somewhere inside of me, I was hoping to find some major purpose for my life, which the enemy seemed to want to derail. Thoughts flashed across my mind: dreams and potential adventures in ministry, the journey to America and the obstacles we had encountered along the way. After a few moments, I found enough inner silence to hear the answer. What I heard was not what I expected. As I pondered Bill's question, a thought came to my mind that had never occurred to me before. To my knowledge, there had never been three generations of Manwaring men alive at the same time. My father never knew his grandfather, I never knew my father's father, and my sons never knew my father. My eldest son at that time was married but without children. As I told Bill my answer, he and I both knew somehow that this was it. My cancer was the enemy's attempt to continue a pattern of a broken family line. If the enemy can rob every generation of the wealth of former generations, he will keep us in a perpetual cycle of fatherlessness. That state is the curse that Malachi wrote about: *"He will restore the hearts of the fathers* to their children and the hearts of the children to their fathers, so that I will not come and smite the earth with a curse" (Mal. 4:6).

To have three generations of Manwaring men alive at the same time became my *raison d'être*, my reason to be! Family, at that moment, became my reason to fight and is now an even greater reason to be alive. A few days after my conversation with Bill, James, my eldest son, called me from the UK and told me that he and his wife were about to start trying for a baby. He did not know about my encounter in Bill's office; he simply thought that the news would encourage me. Their decision to start a family was not without its challenges, and some health issues would need to be removed, but James wanted me to know that I was to live for the next generation, and that he was going to play his part in making that a reality.

When I shared this message as a sermon for the first time in May 2008, I promised the church that one day I would stand on that same platform with my son and my grandson and break a family curse. I would only have to wait 15 months to fulfill that promise. In August 2009, James, his wife Amy, my grandson Aidan, and I stood together on that platform and declared that generational curses had been broken from our family and would be broken from others as well. It was, and always will be, one of the best days of my life.

Family is a bigger idea than most of us have been raised to believe. Perhaps we have taken it for granted, or, because of so many broken family lines, we have not fully embraced God's picture of family. Sometimes, out of self-preservation, we reduce our value for families, especially when we observe the inadequacy of our own. We think we can somehow protect ourselves from the pain of knowing that we have less of something that is of such high value to God. Family really is God's big idea: His dream, His view of what is beautiful.

Life began as a perfect family in a perfect garden, and it ends with a perfect wedding. His government is a family model. His ways are love and relationship. His desires are unity and oneness among His kids, and between them and Himself. I sometimes teach that a large part of finding your purpose in life is to discover what is beautiful to you. I believe that the tri-une Godhead did just that. They saw beauty in their small family, and they purposed all of their resources to create one big, beautiful family. The purpose of government on the earth is too often lost amidst the management and maintenance of an organization or nation. But the purpose of government is the creation of society, of family, where every member plays their part in fulfilling the vision of that society.

One of my favorite verses in the Bible is Isaiah 9:7. It is an inspiring verse, but its true meaning relies on the correct definition of the words contained within it. The verse begins: *"There will be no end to the increase of His government."* If government is management and maintenance, then this may be the most boring verse in the Bible. But if government is about relationships, particularly healthy ones that, together, form a society in which each member can reach his or her fullest potential, then it is perhaps one of the top ten most motivational verses.

Further along in Isaiah 9, we read of justice and righteousness, two attributes I have written about in my book *What on Earth is Glory?* But I will briefly explain here that these two words have also been misunderstood. *Righteousness* is often represented as a set of rules, which we are required to conform to. And *justice* is believed to be the punishment for not keeping those rules. But righteousness is, however, an invitation to be like God, an assignment given to us by the apostle Paul in Ephesians 5:1. Justice, I would like to suggest, is everything we need in order to accept that invitation. We are justified—an old engineering term that was reborn for a computer age to describe the alignment of the text on a page. We are lined up with the original standard, which is perfect relationship with our heavenly family: God the Father, God the Son, and God the Holy Spirit.

Start to look for your "reason to be" as it relates to this greatest assignment of all: to create a family on earth that mirrors heaven's family. The reason for nearly every deficit of our souls can be found in the deficits that exist in our earthly relationships—father wounds, as they are often called, or the wounds of a mother or even a friend.

I recently watched the extraordinary movie *127 Hours*, along with a documentary that was released after the Hollywood film. It is the grueling story of a man whose arm gets trapped under a rock while he is hiking. His only option for survival is to sever his arm with a small pocketknife. He lives to tell the tale. In the documentary, this young man shares that at one point during the 127 hours that he was trapped, in some form of hallucination, he saw a young boy, a son. He described that he had, in part, found strength to do the unthinkable and save his own life through the realization that he was to live for a generation that was yet to be born. By the time the documentary was made, he was married and his wife had given birth to a son. His story—though much more graphic—seems to parallel mine. He found the most valuable vision for the future: a son and a family.

For that very same reason I found purpose to fight. And for that reason this book is dedicated to Aidan James Manwaring. He is a first of many whose very existence breaks a curse. So many times in my life I have fallen short of the understanding that the core purpose of life is relationship. In the last chapter of the book of Job is a simple verse that can be easily missed: *"After this, Job lived 140 years, and saw his sons and his grandsons, four generations"* (Job 42:16). What an incredible way to close this book. A man who had lost everything at the beginning of the story ends his life with the great reward of four generations of family alive together at the same time.

Two years after my surgery, I was preparing to preach a message at Bethel. The evening before I was meant to preach, Sue told me that she had a vision of Aidan as a grown man, having just had his first son. And in the vision, we were there to go into the room and see our great-grandson. Sue knew nothing of the content of the sermon I was preparing. I was getting ready to preach about the restoration of Job's family, the gift of generations, and the ways in which God had restored life to me both during and since my surgery. I would call that message "Restored Fortunes."

Chapter 11

Restored Fortunes

"The Lord restored the fortunes of Job…" (Job 42:10).

The word *fortune* has typically been associated with luck or gambling, probably due to common usage in reference to lotteries and casinos. Fortune has, therefore, always been representative to me of something outside of the way we should live life in relationship with God. That ended one day when I was reading the book of Job, the tale of a man's tragic life and the failure of his friends to help him. However, when you look past the tragedy and the failure of his friends, you will find a life that ends surprisingly well.

Many times I have found a rich depth in the book of Job, a book that theologians believe to be the oldest in the Bible. It contains the great statement: *"I know that my Redeemer lives"* (Job 19:25), which is both a truth and a prophetic cry. This statement is then fulfilled in the last chapter of the book, as God restores the fortunes of Job with a double measure (see Job 42:10). That is the work of a Redeemer! However, that declaration is but one example of many that reveals the character of the man, Job. God described him as an upright man, not a description commonly given in the Bible, yet one that he was certainly worthy of (see Job 1:8).

The beginning of Job contains a devastating account, the details of which are hard to understand. The events and story that follow the dramatic deaths of Job's family show his incredible character—character, which, I have no doubt, is the reason his fortunes were eventually restored to him. To give but one example: after hearing the news of the tragic loss of his entire family and livelihood, Job "bowed low and worshiped" (see Job 1:21). This was the posture of his life. He was a worshiper who would not blame God or agree with the men who eventually came to "comfort" him. The Bible says that Job did not sin or blame God (see Job 1:22). These characteristics of worship and living completely unoffended at God paved the way for his life to be fully restored to him.

The week before I had my surgery, at the close of a worship service, I announced to the church that I had prostate cancer and I would be having surgery on Good Friday. I asked the congregation to do something for me—to stand and worship with me. The lesson of worshiping in the midst of what we don't understand is foundational. Bill Johnson taught me this, but I have no idea who taught Job. Job is possibly the oldest book in the Bible; his story, therefore, one of the oldest in the Bible. And there, on the pages of this ancient book, is the story of a man who knew exactly what to do when his life circumstances went beyond his understanding. He fell to the ground and he worshiped.

I know that some of you who are reading this are in the midst of difficult circumstances. Although maybe not as difficult as Job's, whatever you are facing is likely hell on earth for you right now. These are the experiences of life when we think to ourselves, "I've seen it on the TV, other people have been through it, but now it is visiting my house." I was in that position with cancer. I'd been around it. I was a nurse for five years, prayed for people battling cancer throughout my entire Christian life, and then it suddenly visited my home. I want to release hope to you, that your fortunes will be restored just like Job's were. There is no circumstance—Job's circumstances are off every chart that I have ever seen—that is beyond our God. Job's entire family, community, livelihood, and income were all destroyed, but he knew two things to do: worship and not blame God. We likely and rightfully associate grace with the New Testament. However, this potentially oldest story in the Bible is played out in the context of grace.

At the close of the story, after Job's friends had failed to help him out of his situation, God then told those friends to go and visit Job. God could have legitimately dealt with them another way, but instead He told them that He would treat them according to Job's faithfulness if they would offer up sacrifices (see Job 42:8). That is grace; pure, undiluted grace! The incredible truth revealed here is that if we walk faithfully, walk in worship and walk forward, and don't blame God when things go wrong, then we are able to allow other people to step under the covering of our lives and experience the breakthrough that we have fought for and won. Another way of looking at it is that in as much as we overcome, we are able to give an impartation of overcoming to others. As you walk through different seasons of your life and allow other people to come under the covering of your victories, you reveal Jesus, the Great Overcomer! He overcame the grave and death, and therefore covers us and enables us to walk in victory. If He can restore Job's fortunes, He can restore anybody's fortunes.

Job had quite a lot to begin with. We read in the first chapter of the book that he was the wealthiest man in the entire East. Yet, at the end of his life, he gets two-fold in return, except when it comes to his family. God restored to him seven sons and three daughters, exactly the same as at the beginning of the story. Incidentally, I believe that God didn't need to give Job 14 sons and 6 daughters, double what he originally had. You can't replace people and you don't need to. But you can always add to relationships. You see, there is an eternal nature to the human soul. When God restored to Job seven sons and three daughters, He was adding to the family that Job already had, one that was no longer on earth.

Then, at the very end of the book, we read that Job died an old man and full of days (see Job 42:17). This is my plan, to die an old man and full of days. To me, full of days means fully satiated. It means lying on your deathbed with no regrets. It means that you got everything there was to get out of life, and you gave everything there was to give. I believe that there is a prophetic message in this as well. By way of an interpretation, I believe the message is that this is what a restored life looks like; this is what a restored community looks like.

The sequence of restoration in Job's life provides a revelation of the standard to aim for when seeking restoration in our own lives. Firstly, we see that all of Job's brothers, all of his sisters, all who had known him before, turn up at his doorstep, and there is reconciliation, comfort, celebration, and generosity. That's what community does. Covenant community celebrates with each other. One of the main characteristics of Job's fortunes having been restored is the reconciliation of relationships.

As I shared in a previous chapter, when I had my inner healing session (Sozo) before my surgery, I said to Dawna De Silva, who was leading the session, "I want to make sure there's nothing in me, because I have got prostate cancer and I've read *A More Excellent Way* by Henry Wright, and sometimes this cancer is associated with lust and pornography and stuff like that."

Dawna looked straight at me and said, "You are clean." I've had a couple of Sozos from her before, so she knew me pretty well. She then said that I had a "supplanter spirit." When Dawna said that, I knew it was the right word; so after she left my house, I wrote an e-mail to my older sister. Dawna may have known that I have an older sister, but what she didn't know is that I hadn't spoken to her for 19 years. Sue and I had done the best we could, everything we knew to do in those 19 years, to try and restore the relationship.

In my e-mail to my sister, I told her about the inner healing session and Dawna's revelation. I then apologized for stealing her relational birthright when I was born—which I believed to be the interpretation of the word. Obviously, I was a baby when this happened, and I didn't actually sit up in my crib and say, "Hi, now I'm stealing your birthright!" I simply had to show up on the planet. But because of some comments made about my sister and about my birth, and because of other circumstances involving our relatives, my birth robbed her of her birthright. My sister wrote back to me and told me that she cried when she read my apology. My wife and I had often discussed wanting my sister to come back into our lives, so long as she didn't want to dig up the past. When my sister wrote, she said that she wanted to come visit us, but under one circumstance: that we wouldn't dig up the past. That was all we needed to hear.

In September of 2008, my sister came and stayed in our house, and it was the easiest thing in the world.

I felt fully restored. I just have one sister, so all of my sisters and brothers are restored to me: 100 percent. We need to learn to live in expectation of this type of restoration. An experience like mine should be the norm, the thing that we're going after: restored, reconciled relationships.

When relationships come into order, it is the government of heaven encountering earth. As we previously discovered, the government of heaven is God the Father, God the Son, and God the Holy Spirit: three in one. So perfect in their loyalty to each other, their honor for each other, their understanding of each other's purpose, and so secure in the identity of each one, that you can glance at the three and think you only saw one. They are three in one and one in three; they are relationship defined and personified.

Jesus lived, died, and rose from the grave that we might be restored in relationship to each other and the Father. When you have relationships restored, you have government established; and when you have government established, there's no end to increase. Order always brings increase. God created man and woman: the perfect order of relationship. The primary structure of government on earth was a man and a woman who married. And what happens when that order is put in place? Increase! And so it was with Job. The Lord blessed the latter days of Job more than his early days, and Job ended up with 14,000 sheep, 6,000 camels, 1,000 yoke of oxen, and 1,000 female donkeys. Expect increase!

That order brings increase is a foundational principle according to the way God created this planet. He told us to be fruitful and multiply (see Gen. 1:28). Our planet is designed for increase. Earth's population has been steadily increasing to the current population of 7 billion, and it will continue to increase. There is a momentum occurring on this planet, a momentum of increase.

Seven more sons and three more daughters were born to Job. That is increase. Then the Bible says this: *"He named the first Jemimah, and the second Keziah, and the third Keren-happuch"* (Job 42:14). There are no sons named. It is rare to find only the daughters named in the Bible. Could it be that a characteristic of a society in which the fortunes of the richest man are fully restored is that the daughters are named as heirs of the inheritance? Could it be that one of the characteristics of redemption is equality and identity?

I don't know if you have ever studied the word *redemption*, but it is a big word. Interestingly, the word *redeemer* only appears in the Old Testament. I have a message that I jokingly call, "There is no redeemer in the New Testament." The word nearest to redeemer in the New Testament is *archegos*, from which we get the word *architect*. A fuller meaning of *redeemer*, as used in the Old Testament, is "the one who pays the ransom, builds the pathway to take you from captivity to freedom, builds the city where you will live, and remains as sovereign ruler and protector."[1] Like I said, redeemer is a big word! The Greek *archegos*, used four times in the New Testament, has a similar meaning. Each time it is used, it refers to a person. Its most notable use is in Hebrews 12:2, *"Looking unto Jesus, the author* [archegos] *and finisher of our faith"* (NKJV). It was not just Job who experienced redemption, but his daughters experienced it as well.

Some time ago, I heard a man preach a message that the names of these three daughters paint a picture of the end-time Bride of Christ. *Jemimah* means "as fair as the day," *Keziah* means "a fragrant aroma or total consecration," and *Keren* means "rays of light" or "child of beauty and purity." That's the Bride I want to be part of. I want to be part of the Bride that's as fair as the day, that's about total consecration, that's most beautiful in all the land, that is known for rays of light, that is a child of beauty, and is known for purity. That's the Bride He's coming back for. He's coming back for a Bride that is ready. He's coming back for a pure, spotless, beautiful Bride! And I believe that it's going to take our women to help get the Bride ready.

The Church, the Bride of Christ, has not always been an attractive role model to the world. The

Church has not always been a role model that is as fair as the day, pure, a child of beauty, or totally consecrated. Jesus said we are supposed to be known for love and unity (see John 13:35). And we've been too often known for protestation and disunity. But here is the good news: I think that when we put our women in their rightful place, we are going to begin to see the Church return to its rightful place.

The picture of a society in which Job's fortunes are fully restored looks like this: the women are given a name, and in that context, the Bride becomes beautiful. It says clearly that *"in all the land no women were found so fair as Job's daughters"* (Job 42:15). I don't know about you, but I believe the Bride of Christ should be the greatest organization on the planet. There should be people lined up, coming to get counsel and hear wisdom and be part of the Bride of Christ. There should be none other like the Bride of Christ, and we're going to get to that place because He is Redeemer.

It is not just in the naming of the daughters that we see the Bride of Christ in the story of Job. After he names them, we learn that *"their father gave them inheritance among their brothers"* (Job 42:15). It seems that somewhere in history we lost this. We generally have a culture where the males inherit first, but Job, as I have said, in potentially the oldest book in the Bible, gave the daughters inheritance among their brothers. Not only that, but this inheritance was apparently given before Job died. This may have been similar to New Testament examples of inheritance. In the days of the apostle Paul, the culture of inheritance was roughly this: you were a child until the age of 12, at which time there would be a ceremony denoting entry into manhood. From age 12 to 30, or thereabouts, you would serve as an apprentice, and at around age 30, you would be given your inheritance. The inheritance given at 30 often looked like your father setting you up in a family business and building you a house or adding an extension on the family home for you to bring your bride to. And that's the way it's meant to be: equality is *given*. Notice it's not equality that's taken, it's not equality that's fought for, it's equality that is given.

After giving his inheritance, Job lived 140 years, seeing his sons and his grandsons for four generations: *"And Job died, an old man and full of days"* (Job 42:17). A few years ago, Martin Scott, a British prophet, visited Bethel Church and gave us a prophetic word about fathers who raise fathers, not just sons. He spoke about the importance of creating a culture of three generations of fathers living and serving together. But I want to add one to it. I want to add the fourth generation because there are four generations mentioned in Job. I believe Job is a model of what a redeemed community looks like, and it includes four generations.

We are meant to live in four generations of blessing, to live with fathers all around us. In the natural, I should have a father and a father-in-law, four grandfathers, and eight great-grandfathers in my life. I should have those kinds of relationships because that's what blessing looks like. As it is, I don't have any of those. My life journey is like this: there were two generations of Manwaring men alive at the same time. Then, when I was 15, it was reduced to one generation. When I was 25, I bumped it up to two generations. At age 50, I came under an attack of prostate cancer that tried to stop there ever being three generations of Manwaring men alive at the same time. But the devil lost that one, and now there are three generations of Manwaring men alive today. I'm relationally deficit in my life. I have a sister, but I have no brothers, daughters, or fathers. In fact, because of that, my mother and my wife never had fathers-in-law. The only reason I'm reasonably together is because I have somebody who redeems everything! He gives everything back. And the same is true for you.

I'm privileged to have those in my life that I can call daughters and who call me father. He restores all things. When God restores fortunes, there is a clear picture, a specific kind of community that we get to live in, and this is what He wants to declare over us. This is how He wants us to live. He wants us to know that when we put relationships in order, He brings increase. He wants us to see that there is a place of inheritance for women. Not only that, but He wants us to see that the Bride of Christ has feminine qualities and, more importantly, needs women to help us run it, lead it, build it, and show the world what the Bride of Christ really looks like. He wants us to see that inheritance is a big deal; it plays a big part in the way we do life. Inheritance isn't meant to be passed on at death. It is meant to be for now; it's meant to be something that we apprentice for. We are meant to find ourselves proven capable before our parents and receive our inheritance so that they can watch us run with it. They should have the privilege of seeing what we will do with what we've been given and not wait until they sit in the great cloud of witnesses to see how well we have lived and passed on all that they've given us.

This, to me, is a picture of what God intended our community to look like. He's coming back for a Bride that's prospering, one that's in relational order. He's coming back for a Bride whose women, as well as the men, have a name. He's coming back for a Bride whose women share the inheritance and who has fathers everywhere you look. What do fathers do? They release identity and purpose, and they provide security. Fathers also provide protection. That's what we are in need of on planet earth today. The world is crying out for a place to go to find identity, purpose, security, and protection.

When we experience difficult times, what is one of the things that we most often say? "I want justice. Give me some justice, God." Do you know what justice looks like? Job 42. Justice doesn't happen, by and large, in the courts of our land. That's called law. My definition of the purpose of justice, as laid out for us in the Bible, is the restoration of relationships. What happened to Job at the end of his book is justice. It is justice fully defined. Whoever you are, whatever the circumstances of your life, justice for you is His goal and His plan. If you feel you've been living in Job chapters 1 to 41, there is a Job 42 for your life.

I believe that we need to start declaring justice because the curse is undone through blessing. The four-generational curse is going to be undone by a four-generational blessing. Jesus became a curse so that we wouldn't have to. We are blessed. You were born to inherit a blessing; and when a father blesses you, you immediately receive a double blessing. You already have one blessing just by who you are, just by entering this world. As soon as the fathers and mothers in your life begin to bless you, you step straight into double blessing.

Perhaps my favorite verse in the book of Job is 5:16, which is beautifully turned into song by William Matthews in "Hope's Anthem": "So the helpless has hope, and unrighteousness must shut its mouth." It is a deep truth that when the helpless find hope, not an answer, not even the promise of one, but hope—an earnest expectation of good—unrighteousness is silenced. If unrighteousness is silenced, there can only be one consequence: the voice of righteousness can be heard. Job found that hope in a helpless place, and unrighteousness was silenced and his fortunes were restored. I encourage you to take this picture of restored fortunes, and with it, find hope for yourself and for others.

Endnote

1. James Strong, *Strong's Exhaustive Concordance of the Bible.*

Chapter 12

Become a Kiss

In the more extreme circumstances of life, the simple things not only become profound, but when it comes to words spoken or acts of kindness, simple is often the most powerful. Perhaps that is why in Matthew 25, Jesus says that He will judge nations on the basis of whether or not they have fed the hungry, clothed the naked, given water to the thirsty, and visited the prisoners and the sick. By providing a list of simple activities, He enables everyone to engage in life. All of us have the ability to give a cup of water to someone needing it, but not all of us can aspire to being the president of a nation. Each one of us has the opportunity to be profound and powerful. It is just likely that our powerful act will be delivered in a simple package.

Jesus paints an incredible picture in Matthew 25, the backdrop of which is the glory of heaven. First, He likens the kingdom of heaven to ten virgins, five who were prepared and five unprepared. He then likens the kingdom of heaven to a man who entrusts the increase of his estate to the faithfulness of his servants. Through His parables, Jesus leaves us with no doubt as to the value system of heaven. But right when we think the story is over, the picture has been painted, He asks us, "Before you knew what heaven valued, did you learn to recognize Me on earth in the elemental lesson of caring for the least?"

We might not be "the least," but during our journey, Sue and I received a profound experience expressed through a simple act of kindness. It happened on Easter Sunday, 2008. Sue and I love Easter. We got engaged on Easter Sunday, 1977, and married on Easter Saturday, 1979. In 2008, however, we were in the midst of our worst Easter Sunday, when a friend stepped into our lives. That day, Sue had thought at one point that I had died or, at the very least, that I would need a pacemaker. I had experienced a catalogue of unprofessional and incompetent nursing and medical care, not, I hasten to add, by my surgeon. Sue was definitely in need of some rest, but she had decided that she was not leaving me in the hospital alone. She had good reason to want to stay.

Instead of the expected second-day return home after surgery, I had been moved to a cardiac ward and, to be honest, we had a very limited understanding as to why I was there. I had no doubt that many in that ward needed more intense care than I did. After they moved me to the ward, Sue and I were left to fend for ourselves, staring at a portable pacemaker at the end of the bed. I don't think anyone knew what was going on.

Late that night, Kevin Dedmon arrived to visit me. It was perfect timing, but it was no ordinary visit. Kevin, increasingly well known for treasure hunts and bringing the supernatural with laughter, joy fests, and short, sharp interventions, arrived as a friend on a mission. That night he became famous in our family. He had heard reports of my "critical" condition during the Easter morning service. That service is famous for a message that Bill preached that day entitled, "I Want My Knife Back." (I believe he has received more testimonies from that one message than any other.) I wasn't there to hear it, but I did need something back: I wanted my life back! Kevin came to release a healing anointing, but he quickly realized that Sue was exhausted, so he decided that he was not leaving until she was settled. The tone of his voice and actions indicated that he would stay all night if necessary.

It is hard to put into words what this meant to us. Kevin pastored and fathered us, and, since we had no family other than our sons in town, he became the family that Sue needed at that moment. He started hunting the hospital for the most comfortable recliner chair and rearranged the ward furniture. His fearless character was not concerned with the opinion of the hospital staff as much as with Sue's comfort. To be honest, 25 years from now I may not remember the details of Kevin's preaching, but I will never forget his redesign of Sue's sleeping arrangements that Easter Sunday of 2008. Kevin became a kiss from a good God. His visit was a timely intervention, and his capacity to recognize our needs allowed the love of heaven to bring rest to my exhausted wife.

During my journey, the reality was that many people were the carriers of kisses from God. I am sure the road my family and I traveled really does justify the use of the sometimes-overused phrase, "I had grace for it." My favorite definition of grace is from Philip Yancey's book *What's So Amazing About Grace?* He says that *grace* is "God's empowering presence." For me, grace is best defined after the event, when, as you look back, you know that you couldn't do it again were it not for grace.

Grace manifested in three primary areas in my life during that season: the grace to live a certain lifestyle, the grace to recognize the kisses that came directly from God, and the grace that was the kisses brought to me by brothers and sisters. It is this third point that I want to emphasize throughout this chapter. I want to encourage every person who reads this book to live his or her life looking for the opportunity to become a kiss. It often requires the impromptu response to an internal prodding in order to recognize and be the kiss that someone needs. You are the means through which heaven can touch earth. Jesus became flesh, and it is as if every day there is an opportunity for heaven to become flesh over and over again. The incarnation goes on; it wasn't a one-time event. It was the event that would empower us all, for all time, to be Jesus to someone else.

I love Heidi Baker's life message of stopping for "the one." She and her husband, Rolland, missionaries and church planters in Mozambique, live their lives according to the principle that our purpose here on earth is to stop for the one person that God has placed in front of us, the one person who needs a touch of heaven. Each one of us, even if our "one" is not among the orphans of the Third World, has an opportunity to live our lives selflessly by stopping for the one that God places along our path. While what you have to offer may feel like only a small step, for the recipient it may feel more like you came an extra 10,000 miles! I had an experience like that, and I know that the deliverer of that kiss had no idea that her simple action would have a dramatic impact on my life.

It was on my worst day, prior to surgery, that I received this amazing kiss. I was sitting in my office at the church that morning, wondering where my breakthrough was. But more than that, I was wondering whether or not I was truly a supernatural minister of the gospel. I had read my Bible that morning, and there, in my handwriting, next to the verse I was reading, I had written a quote of Bill's: "If you are not a supernatural minister of the gospel, then you are not a minister at all." That quote seemed so right when I first heard it, but at that moment, in my unhealed state, it felt personal, and I began to question my call. Should I resign? I know that many have sat in my same position. I have known church leaders who pursue the supernatural while at the same time struggling with a terminal illness. Sitting in that place requires an incredible faith in God to keep pressing in for the personal breakthrough while leading the church to supernatural breakthrough. It is a double responsibility. The men and women I have seen walk through that are truly my heroes.

I believe that the journey to breakthrough may include a valid moment of questioning regarding call or purpose. But for those of us pursuing the supernatural, this doubt or fear likely has its origins in the enemy's heart. There is no doubt the enemy will try to cause us to give up in the face of adversity, knowing that it is at that very place in the battle when our greatest strength is revealed. Prior to my illness, I had struggled with whether or not I was a supernatural minister of the gospel. In fact, I have lived much of my life through the lens of comparison, and I have never won a contest yet. I have often sat under the ministry of healing evangelists and berated myself for my lack of supernatural or evangelistic impact on the world around me. It is definitely a mistake to live life comparing oneself to others. The enemy wants us to compare ourselves to others and thus disqualify ourselves from the race. But the opposite is what he is really afraid of: that we see who we really are and, because of that, we disqualify the enemy.

For me, I am sure the enemy was the origin of my temptation to resign. That morning, after wondering whether or not I should even be doing what I was doing, I tried to occupy myself, and so I walked to my office mailbox and collected an unassuming envelope. Here, at my lowest moment, I received the greatest encouragement.

Six months before, I had ministered in Texas at a conference. During the afternoon session, a denominational pastor's wife brought her husband to me for prayer. All she told me was that her husband had lost hope of seeing revival in his denomination. I prayed for them—nothing very special happened—and then, to be honest, I quickly forgot the event ever took place. Sitting in my office, six months later, I opened a thank you card from that minister's wife, Amy. In the card, she told me that she had taken notes of my prayer, turned them into a series of declarations, and given them to their intercessors on her return from the conference. The declarations had to do with revival in their denomination, signs and wonders every month of the year, and unity in their city. Amy wrote that since that day they have seen a tumor disappear from behind an eye, a blind eye open, and metal plates disappear from a lady's shoulder. I sat in my office, with tears in my eyes, as I told myself that I *am* a supernatural minister of the gospel. That card changed my journey, not just through cancer, but into the next season of my life as well. Amy was, to me, like the one leper who returned to give thanks. She was a kiss from a good God! Thank you, Amy.

We have, it seems, made life too complicated. We may think that we need to minister in a particular way. But sometimes a simple prompting that connects us to the heart of God, which we then carry to another human being, may very well be as complicated as it gets when it comes to changing a moment or even a life. I experienced many such moments on my journey, and all of them contained, for the individual delivering them, the option of ignoring their inner prompting. Yet an e-mail, a phone call, or even an old-fashioned letter may be the very simple means of releasing one of God's kisses to a fellow traveler.

We are ambassadors of Jesus Christ, His representatives here on earth. As it is sometimes said, "You may be the only Jesus someone encounters today." I often share a message about glory—particularly the glory that we carry. Our glory is to reveal, reflect, or point to God's nature, power, and attributes. That means that even the simple fruits of the Spirit have a glory as they point to the nature and attributes of God. The daily expression of the fruits of the Spirit begins with love, the simplest yet most profound message of all.

Loving ourselves, which often means not comparing ourselves to others, but embracing who He made us to be—and our gifts and calling—is central to our ability to love our neighbors. Jesus commanded that we love our neighbors as ourselves (see Matt. 22:34-40). Yet loving ourselves may be our single toughest assignment during our lives here on earth. If we do not love ourselves, we sell our neighbors short. If we, as I have too often done, spend too long comparing our gift to the gifts of others, then we will dilute that gift, identity, and godly confidence, and may miss the prompting to use our gift to release kisses to others. As we learn to love ourselves and the gifts and fruits that we carry with us, we will enter others' lives with a confidence that we can make a difference.

The word *worship* in the New Testament is often a translation of the Greek word *proscineo*, which means, "to lean towards as if to kiss."[1] As we learn to value Jesus more and more, we are drawn closer and closer to Him as if leaning in to offer a reverent kiss. Perhaps this is what Jesus meant in Matthew 25. As we learn to recognize Him in others, we start to understand His (and their) worth. And, it is as if, through our actions of love, we lean in to offer a kiss.

Endnote

1. James Strong, *Strong's Exhaustive Concordance of the Bible.*

Chapter 13

Whispering Shame

I was taken by surprise, soon after my diagnosis, by the introduction into my psyche, of the awareness of shame. I don't believe it had an exact time of entry, but suddenly I knew it was there. It was an uninvited, intermittent companion, and eventually a target, as I began to recognize this energy-sapping enemy. But shame, like fear and even jealousy, is one side of a larger picture.

Fear, for instance, is a normal and required response to threatening circumstances. The image of living in Florida—or some other alligator-infested location—with a predator at the door, will cause the flight or fight system of our bodies to be activated. But if you never open another door again, then you have become, as Peter says, *"frightened by any fear"* (1 Pet. 3:6). Fear is designed to protect us from harm, but if we aren't careful, it will lock us into responses that keep us imprisoned and prevent us from living in the freedom designed for us by our Creator.

Likewise, we read and come to know that our God is a jealous God (see Ex. 20:5). This describes His desire for us, which releases a desire in us to serve only Him and no other gods. But the other side of jealousy is an emotion that caused Lucifer to be cast out of heaven's glory and, from then until time ends, that has become one of the core enemies of man's heart. Jealousy, which was designed to draw us to God, will draw us away from God as we envy others instead of seeking Him.

So, too, is the picture double-sided when it comes to our potential to feel shame. Shame was given to make us aware of right and wrong. However, when attached to us, albeit by a lie related to something that happened or is happening (and not always something we have done wrong), shame is the thing which covers us with a veneer that keeps us from the hand and mercy of God. In Genesis, after the fall, it is recorded that Adam hid (see Gen. 3:8). He didn't hide from God but from the presence of God. Shame was designed as a prompting, but when it becomes a garment we wear or that is put on us, it does the very thing it was designed to prevent: it hides us from the presence of God and others.

Having met my shame with a diagnosis of cancer, I began to find others who felt similar shame for something they had also not done or caused. Shame can proliferate even in the healthiest of environments. The relationship between diet, exercise, and illness, for example, is gaining more ground, and rightfully so. That same relationship, however, can insidiously be converted into a source of self-criticism, leading to shame. It can easily become a thought in your head that, if you had only lived right, you wouldn't be sick. In this move of God that we are a part of, we are learning a lot about how our thoughts can lead to illness, an idea made popular by Henry Wright in his book *A More Excellent Way.* Once again, shame can stealthily multiply as we think to ourselves that we may have, by our behaviors and thoughts, contributed to our disease.

I was surprised to discover how common an experience like mine really was. Added to my diet and thought-life was the surprise that, even in a culture where supernatural healing is a foundational belief, there is another cause of shame. When we passionately believe in healing—and that we will be healed—but it doesn't come as we expect or believe it will, shame can come instead. And that shame prevents us from experiencing the fullness of relationship with the One who bore our sorrow, sickness, sins, and shame!

After being thrown into this complex world of whispering, hidden shame, I realized that this was a part of the fall. The moment Adam ate of the fruit of the tree, his response was to hide. His God-given conscience, which should have prevented him from eating the fruit, instead became the response that caused him to hide from the One who alone is able to forgive. That response is echoed by every one of us who foolishly hide the things we are ashamed of from an all-seeing, all-knowing God. We will see that replayed over and over if we allow shame to be our hiding place.

I began to discover that the greatest way to attack shame is through authenticity. If I am real with God, others, and myself, then shame is exposed and removed, and I can let God know exactly where I am. Authenticity belongs to the kingdom: *"Therefore, confess your sins to one another"* (James 5:16). Shame, as a condition, belongs to the religious spirits that will do all they can to keep us from an authentic relationship with God. In fact, shame belongs to the same spirit that caused the Pharisees to invent rituals that would hide sinful behavior. Jesus addressed them, telling them that the cup was clean on the outside but not the inside (see Matt. 23:25). He came and invited us to confess our sins so that we could be washed and cleansed and our access to God be fully realized. His message was clear. The first Adam hid, but the second Adam removed any reason to hide.

I was recently an emcee at a conference at Bethel, and one morning of the event I received a word of knowledge while in the shower. The word stayed with me all day. When the evening meeting came, I shared with the audience about how I had received a word that morning of people in the crowd who were struggling with suicidal thoughts. There was absolutely no response from any of the 350 people in the room. So I told the audience that if the word applied to them, to wait for another word and then stand up so that they wouldn't be embarrassed. I passed the microphone down the line, and the ministry team shared other words of knowledge. Once I had passed the microphone, a young woman came up to me and encouraged me, saying that the word about suicide was correct. I knew it was because I really could feel it. I remembered walking through prisons after there had been a suicide, and I recognized the tangible feeling in my spirit. As I listened to the other words of knowledge, I began to realize that by giving people permission to not respond to my word, I had unintentionally released an atmosphere associated with shame. I had actually told people to hide when what was required was a moment of transparency.

The microphone was returned to me, and many people were now standing in response to the words of knowledge. I knew what I had to do; I needed to undo the atmosphere I had created by sharing my own journey of shame. In front of the conference guests, I shared my story of the shame of prostate surgery, and the feeling that everyone would think me unable to have an intimate relationship with my wife post-surgery. It was, in reality, not many years ago that the only outcome to such surgery was the inability to be intimate. Now, with the genius of nerve-sparing surgery, it doesn't have to be that way! As I ended my story, I gave another call for those feeling suicidal. Almost immediately, a young man wearing a bright blue t-shirt walked to the front of the room. His simple action of transparency changed the atmosphere. Twelve to 15 more people responded to the word and came forward into the light of transparency where their healing could be received.

The first time I publicly shared my cancer story, I ended by addressing shame. I can't tell you if this would have been the case had I lost my ability to make love to my wife. I do know that she and I had to face that possibility, and that alone has given me a place of understanding. As Isaiah 43 states, our identity is in Him, not the fire, flood, or storm. We may stink of smoke, be drenched and windswept, but our identity is in Him. Circumstances, life experience, or even roles do not give us our identity. I often think of Jesus in this regard. On earth, He had no earthly father, but He was the perfect Son. He had no earthly sons, but He was the perfect Father. As Servant, Son, and Lover, He that never married shows all men how to love their brides. He brought that identity with Him, beautifully portrayed in Isaiah 9:6: *"For unto us a Child is born, unto us a Son is given; and the government will be upon His shoulder. And His name will be called Wonderful, Counselor, Mighty God, Everlasting Father, Prince of Peace"* (NKJV). He brought His identity with Him!

Shame is destroyed by authenticity and love. It is true in the story of Peter. Peter, who had denied being associated with Jesus and who then went off alone, returned to Jesus by diving into a freezing cold sea and swimming to his Lord. But even after that act of devotion, he had to declare his love for Jesus. Three times Jesus asked him, "Do you love Me?" (see John 21:15-17). It was as if Jesus was asking him, "Peter, are you really back? Or are you still hiding behind words and actions?" Jesus was seeking an authentic response from him.

Shame has allowed the human race to hide from God since Adam. It has created false and temporary sanctuaries built on lies. Shame will create a guard-edness, or even an overconfidence, and either will prevent access to those who could speak truth into our lives—whether friends, family, or God. When Jesus bore our shame, He removed the need to hide. He created a pathway to God where nothing needs to be hidden. In fact, the entire agenda was reversed. The old way was cover-up, and the new way became confession. The old way was to appear flawless, but the new way was to be made flawless. And that is the picture of the Bride in Ephesians, pure and spotless (see Eph. 5:22-33).

As I write, I am conscious of so many aspects of life that can inflict shame on a person. I was privileged to spend 12 weeks working in obstetrics as a student nurse. I watched as some babies literally fell out of their mothers and onto the gurney between antenatal care and the delivery room, while other parents had to endure many obstacles and hurdles before cuddling their newborn. The language and experience of natural childbirth is highly desired, but if a mother has to have a cesarean, she is no less amazing, courageous, or spiritual. Yet, I have met some mothers who have felt shame because they didn't achieve the elusive natural birth.

Sue and I have often discussed breast cancer. No woman wants to lose a breast, but we always knew what we would do if faced with the painful decision of a mastectomy. We have not had to face that, but we know many who have, and they are no less women for it. In fact, they may be more so because of a journey they had to take into what really makes them who they are.

While my journey ended well, it included a trip through the hall of mirrors, which is a trip through shame. The hall of mirrors, for me, was a journey of reflections and lies that bounced back at me, taunting me while I tried to keep my eyes on what is most important: relationship with my identity, relationship with my triune, heavenly family, and with my wife and earthly family. Shame, if left to its own devices, will wreck all of these. In reality, shame is but a gossamer-thin covering, waiting to be ripped off to allow the full glory of who we are to be revealed.

Sometimes, in our desire to find a solution, we can inadvertently inflict shame on others, as someone did when they told me that my diet had caused my cancer. That may or may not be true, but it certainly wasn't helpful! Shame separates, but love connects. And it is love we need, for shame's brother, fear, is lurking, and perfect love will expel him too.

Just recently, my wife, through building relationship with a young woman, had the opportunity to provide an environment in which that young woman could encounter a loving God, a God who would not judge her if surgery was required. There was shame on this young woman, but it quickly left. Through loving counsel, she recognized that she had permission to open doors that had previously been closed to her. She was transformed. Relationship created the opportunity for love's great work of freedom to be accomplished. Her circumstances and diagnosis haven't yet changed, but her positioning with Father, self, and others has changed dramatically.

In the book *The Cross and the Prodigal*, by Kenneth E. Bailey, I learned the historical reason the father ran to his son in the story of the prodigal son. I have heard many messages preached from this biblical story, all of them adding to my perspective, but I had never before heard the following details. The author of this book explains that in the culture of the day, when a son squandered his inheritance, the villagers were permitted to hold a ceremony, called *Kazazah*. This ceremony involved the villagers placing a clay pot at the edge of the village and smashing it in front of the son as a demonstration that he was no longer welcome in that village. He was, in other words, shamed. Bailey goes on to say that the reason the father ran was, quite simply, to get to the son before the villagers did. Before the villagers smashed the clay pot, the mother was permitted to go and kiss the son good-bye, but the father was not. He was required to remain in the house. However, that was not the result of this great story as told from the lips of Jesus. In the telling of this story, He was—as He often did—turning culture on its head.

This portrayal of a prodigal son being hugged, kissed, and welcomed by a father—not submitting to the old law, but to love—must have penetrated the minds and hearts of all who heard. What we now know through Jesus, the people of that day had only a glimpse of in the prophets: that the Father bore our shame through His Son on the cross. In the story of the prodigal son, the father ran and got to his son first, before the villagers could shame and expel him. The son had brought shame on the family and hence, the village, so their goal was to put shame on him forever. But the father would have none of that, and regardless of what was thought of him, he did what no Middle Eastern man should do: hitched up his robe, exposed his legs, and ran. And for the first time after reading this story, I saw something new. I saw that the father bore the shame of his son.

Shame has a ferocious appetite and it will consume whatever it is allowed to consume. However, there is no limit to love. It is continually poured out, bringing hope with it. Isaiah 61 begins with the brokenhearted, the captive, and the prisoner—all circumstances causing shame. However, the chapter ends with a declaration over those very same people: *"Instead of your shame you will have a double portion"* (Isa. 61:7). Heaven's payback for shame is a double portion. Now that is good news.

Chapter 14

Re-Sign

Eighteen months after my surgery, a man came into my office that I had spoken to just once before. This day, however, began our friendship. The first thing he told me was that he had a dream about me. The details of the dream aren't relevant to the story, but it was an accurate dream, confirmed immediately as it related to two other people who had sat in the same seat in my office only days before. Secondly, he gave me the beginning of a prophetic word, which was to become a guiding word for my ministry. It was the third thing he said, however, that was to become a significant part of my healing journey.

As he prayed for me that day, he used the word *resign*, but with an altered emphasis on the word, saying instead, *re-sign*. The significance of that prayer or, more correctly, that single word, could have been easily missed. I have since spoken to the man who prayed for me that day, Steve Witt, about that prayer. He said it was an unprepared prayer and he had no idea of its deep significance. But in that moment, God and Steve got my attention. The dream and the prophetic word prepared me for this simple prayerful exhortation: re-sign.

The journey into and through cancer had some unforeseen elements. One of those was the loss of the top 20 percent of my personal dreams and visions. Those around me would not have noticed that this had occurred. I have always worked hard and am forward thinking in my work. While this was happening, I was still building Global Legacy and working hard, but I had found that in the journey through a life-threatening disease, I had lost something. The loss was mostly subconscious and ventured into my conscious most often when I was shopping, coming in the form of a fleeting thought, somehow appearing when I was thinking about buying clothes. The thought came as a lie that said I wouldn't live long enough to justify the purchase. My long-term vision, it seemed, was affected. I wasn't depressed, and I was fighting all the way, but a subtle reduction in my quality of dream life and forward thinking was evident. I have since come to realize this is not uncommon for those fighting disease or other life-altering circumstances. We were born to look forward, to dream. It's a way of life to be constantly improving things, investing in our thought-life for the sake of ourselves, the world we live in, our children, and our children's children.

Steve's simple prayer gave me the opportunity to re-sign. In other words, I was given a chance to stop accepting my subconscious and to sign up for the long-term vision again. I had no idea, and nor did Steve, that this was a pivotal moment in my healing journey. For one thing, I would be buying shirts again! The spirit of resignation is a serious one, and much of our Western culture is dominated by it. It is, for me, a relative of retirement, which is not a biblical subject apart from the instructions given to the priests to retire in Leviticus. I am not opposed to seeing an end to the nine-to-five, Monday through Friday pace of life. But to retire, to put up one's feet, so to speak, and stop impacting this world? That is not in my thinking. I love the pastors on call and elders at Bethel, some of them serving in their 80s. My own mother in England, at age 89 and 38 years a widow, still visits the sick and the prisoner.

Re-signing is the way of the kingdom; constant upgrades for the next leg of our journey, from glory to glory! Even the word *retire* can be reemphasized as *re-tire*, putting new tires on and enlisting for more miles on our journey. A little while ago, I prayed this re-sign prayer over a man who approached me after a meeting. I gave him a cheap disposable pen, all I had on me at that moment, as a prophetic sign. The next day, he returned and gave me a pen, saying that he noticed I spend more money on my shirts than my pens! I told him that it was buying nice shirts that had raised my awareness of needing to re-sign in the first place. A year later, I sat with him at dinner, a transformed man, full of life and hope, and signed up for a long-term impact on the world and areas where he ministers.

Re-signing is not just an issue for those who are more advanced in years; it is for all of us. I will never forget how, as a young nurse, I took a bone cancer victim across the Whitechapel road to a fast food restaurant. Her leg had been amputated just below the hip and her arm was hurting from using a crutch, so she hopped to get around. Her love for life and expectation of living beyond her disease was evident to all as she hopped and laughed her way across that busy road. She chose to live and not resign, despite the life-threatening and incapacitating disease that attacked her body. Hers was a story that I would see repeated many times in my six months of pediatric nursing at a teaching hospital where only the very sick children came.

The example of the young girl with only one leg is graphic, yet the temptation to give in is likely to be less blatant; the spirit of resignation is a pernicious one. It invades so much of life, causes us to accept what should be challenged, and reduces us to victims instead of being more than conquerors.

The heroes of my life fall into two categories: those who did not let circumstances affect their attitude toward life, and those who went out and changed their circumstances. They are the champions of personal battles and the social reformers. People like Lance Armstrong, and his amazing battle with cancer and successive Tour de France victories, are truly inspirational. When my youngest son, Luke, heard my diagnosis, he ordered a box of yellow Lance Armstrong wristbands that declared "Livestrong." He drew strength from someone whose personal battle had been played out on the world stage with amazing results. He and I have common heroes like Dr. Martin Luther King Jr. and William Wilberforce, these men who rose up and challenged popular belief. They did not resign, and I am sure they had to re-sign many times in their hearts as they entered another arena to battle and abolish the unacceptable faces of racism and slavery.

The victims who rise up and take the ground constantly challenge and inspire me. That is the story of Isaiah 61. This incredible chapter eluded me for years until, one day, I saw that it was the healed, the set free, and the released prisoners who rebuild the ruined city and raise up the former generations. It is not those who have had life handed to them, but those who have faced the greatest challenges of life and won it back. It is the story of Goliath's sword, hidden, waiting to be put back into commission, to be used against the enemy. For the entire time I fought cancer, I had on my mantelpiece a bayonet head from Saddam Hussein's armory in Iraq. A friend had brought it back as a gift for me. It was my prophetic symbol: I will turn against the enemy the sword used against me. This book is part of my sword. Everything I've written here was learned and experienced in the midst of battle, and I will use it to shine light and bring hope to someone else's battle.

As Churchill said during the war: Keep running to the end. Never give in. There is a story of him speaking at Harrow School on October 29, 1941. There was great expectation among the audience, waiting for the speech from the wartime hero and orator. He gave a great speech, but it is most remembered for a simple phrase, which he repeated several times: "Never give in, never give in, never, never, never, never—in nothing, great or small, large or petty—never give in except to convictions of honour and good sense."[1]

Maybe you have never thought of resignation as being from the enemy, and maybe it isn't always, but a *spirit* of resignation certainly is. Not until we can say, "It is finished," and breathe our last, should we resign. Until then, *re-sign*. Look around you. There will be a place for you to use the strength that you have gained in battle and offer it to someone who is in the heat of his or her own.

My friends Mark and Lynette learned to do this during and after their greatest tragedy. Their only son had a terrible brain cancer, a diagnosis which ended in his ultimately going home. As they lived through the unimaginable, we watched them minister to other families in what they thought were worse circumstances. They did not give up in the midst of the fight, nor have they after their loss. When I teach on discovering destiny, I always think of them as an example that sometimes the circumstances outside of our control can have the greatest impact on our destiny. This was certainly true of Lynette. Since her son's death, she has dedicated her life to helping those who are experiencing the trial of watching their child fight cancer. She has published her own book and is now a trained coach. She discovered, in part, in the uncontrollable and unthinkable circumstances of her life, a purpose and a destiny. It will never replace her Matt, for whom she daily longs, but by refusing to resign, she has become one who rebuilds ruined cities out of her own devastation.

Destiny may seem a distant word in the midst of a crisis or test, but there may be clues for your destiny that are learned in such circumstances. I like to call this the "Frodo Factor," after the character in the *Lord of the Rings*. For Frodo, it was picking up and wearing a ring that would lead him on a journey of self-discovery. That ring, and the choice to pick it up, was his means to finding new friends, getting hold of a vision far greater than the one he originally had, and gaining the strength needed to rally armies and fight extraordinary battles. I often like to ask people, "Do you have a 'Frodo Factor'?" Have you awoken one day and found that your plans are in shreds and unforeseen circumstances have invaded your world? Your destiny may not be revealed overnight or immediately—in fact, it rarely is—but, in the midst of your circumstances, there may be great clues to your future successes.

Even before my diagnosis and the subsequent battle with cancer, my wife demonstrated this principle to me and to our family. She led our family to California, and to our present way of life, in the midst of some of her most challenging personal circumstances. She refused to resign; instead she pursued, she re-signed, and she literally began a new life for us all. The history books are full of heroes who re-signed. I invite you now to re-sign, whatever that means for you in this moment. Perhaps you face something that is tempting you to take a more leisurely path through life, when an invitation to get up and climb is staring you in the face. The battle will be in the mind, even though it will likely manifest in the flesh. Your temptation to resign is, in fact, your invitation to write history. And there is grace for it.

Endnote

1. "Selected Speeches of Winston Churchill." *Welcome to Winston-Churchill.org* http://www.winstonchurchill.org/learn/speeches/speeches-of-winston-churchill (Accessed Jan. 27, 2012).

Afterword

At the time of writing this book, I am nearly four years cancer free and entirely grateful to God, Sue, and a great doctor. This has been a season of learning to stay on top of my thoughts and avoiding anything that could introduce irrational doubt. During this time, blood tests every three months have been required, and then celebrated as each clear report has been received. I have aimed to take every opportunity to encourage others along the way. I am especially grateful that my appointments have been more social than medical, as my doctor has enjoyed the opportunity to talk to one of his success stories. We have used our time together to be refreshed, and talk about things like cameras and how God heals with and without doctors.

I have a rather analytical mind, which has been my curse *and* my friend. My mind has often tried to understand why the most incredible miracles, where there is evidence of healing but no explanation other than God, do not make it to the front pages of newspapers. There is, it seems, an entire medical and media world that is either oblivious to these miracles or deceived into believing there is some other explanation. Incredibly, there is even medical language for someone who is raised from the dead. The medical world has ironically used a biblical example to define an inexplicable event, but without giving credit to God. It is called the "Lazarus Syndrome." Those of you reading this are likely to know and believe differently. However, I have concluded that, although I would love to see the before and after x-rays and MRI scans displayed across the screens and pages of the world, even that is unlikely to silence the skeptics.

However, more important than proving wrong the skeptics of the world is revealing who God truly is. If there is one lasting message that I would want to convey from this book, it is the message of His goodness. There will likely be things along your path, as there were along mine, that you do not understand. The task is never to allow those things to obscure the goodness of God. Far better would it be that His goodness would be put on display in our lives. Our journeys should testify that He really is good: goodness is the substance of His being. As for me and my journey, His goodness has enabled three generations of male Manwarings to be alive together. We are especially grateful for this!

One of my family's favorite movies is *Good Will Hunting*. While there are some parts of the movie that may not be family-friendly, there is a profound scene in which the statement is made: "All of us have bad times, they just remind us of the good times we have taken for granted." The Manwarings have been given an opportunity to live out this truth and learn to be thankful for the good things, both great and small, rare and commonplace. We intend to live thankful for the rest of our days.

As I reflect on my journey, I know that it was just the beginning, even if the enemy wanted it to be the end. I am honored to share my story with you and encourage you as you live out your own story. And I know that through you many others will be encouraged too.

About Paul Manwaring

Paul Manwaring is a pastor and a member of the senior management team at Bethel Church in Redding, California. His primary responsibilities are to oversee Global Legacy, an apostolic, relational network of revival leaders, and to equip and deploy revivalists through his oversight of the third-year program in Bethel's School of Supernatural Ministry (BSSM).

Paul truly carries the gift of administration/government and releases that power and wisdom through his Supernatural Strategic Planning Workshops, his itinerant ministry, and his teaching at BSSM. His passion is to see the Bride prepared, glorious sons and daughters revealed, cancer destroyed, and cities transformed as the government of heaven is established on earth.

Paul came to Bethel in 2001, after leaving a career in senior prison management in England. He holds a master's degree in management from Cambridge University and is a registered general and psychiatric nurse.

Visit Paul's website at www.paulmanwaring.com.

IN THE RIGHT HANDS, THIS BOOK WILL CHANGE LIVES!

Most of the people who need this message will not be looking for this book. To change their lives, you need to put a copy of this book in their hands.

> *But others (seeds) fell into good ground, and brought forth fruit, some a hundred-fold, some sixty-fold, some thirty-fold* (Matthew 13:8).

Our ministry is constantly seeking methods to find the good ground, the people who need this anointed message to change their lives. Will you help us reach these people?

> *Remember this—a farmer who plants only a few seeds will get a small crop. But the one who plants generously will get a generous crop* (2 Corinthians 9:6).

EXTEND THIS MINISTRY BY SOWING
3 BOOKS, 5 BOOKS, 10 BOOKS, **OR MORE TODAY,**
AND BECOME A LIFE CHANGER!

Thank you,

Don Nori Sr., Founder
Destiny Image
Since 1982

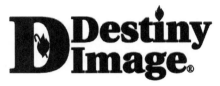

DESTINY IMAGE PUBLISHERS, INC.

"Promoting Inspired Lives."

VISIT OUR NEW SITE HOME AT
WWW.DESTINYIMAGE.COM

FREE SUBSCRIPTION TO DI NEWSLETTER

Receive free unpublished articles by top DI authors, exclusive

discounts, and free downloads from our best and newest books.

Visit www.destinyimage.com to subscribe.

Write to: Destiny Image
              P.O. Box 310
              Shippensburg, PA 17257-0310

Call: 1-800-722-6774

Email: orders@destinyimage.com

For a complete list of our titles or to place an order
online, visit www.destinyimage.com.